Fighting Cancer Naturally

From a Survivor's Perspective

DEDICATION

This book is dedicated, first and foremost, to my friend from Miami, who introduced me to alkaline water. Your introduction sparked my curiosity and led me to explore more about alkaline diets.

I apologize for the delay in completing this book, but God was guiding me through a journey of learning and growth, so I could share better, more valuable information with you. May those who read this and are still with us find benefit in the words within.

CONTENTS

FOREWORD

"Everyone has a physician inside him or her; we just have to help it in its work. The natural healing force within each one of us is the greatest force in getting well. Our food should be our medicine. Our medicine should be our food. But to eat when you are sick is to feed your sickness."

Hippocrates

Prologue

In a world increasingly focused on natural health and wellness, the fight against cancer is evolving. This book, *Fighting Cancer Naturally: From a Survivor's Perspective*, is a culmination of my personal journey and the profound lessons I've learned along the way. It serves as a guide for those navigating the complex terrain of cancer diagnosis and treatment, offering hope and practical strategies for harnessing the power of an alkaline diet.

When I received my cancer diagnosis, I felt as if my world had been turned upside down. The initial shock was overwhelming, accompanied by fear, confusion, and a relentless stream of questions: Why me? What can I do? As I delved into research and explored various treatment options, I discovered the transformative potential of an alkaline diet—a nutritional approach that resonated deeply with me. This wasn't just a diet; it was a pathway to reclaiming my health and nurturing my body in ways I had never imagined.

My motivation for writing this book stems from a desire to share what I've learned with others who find themselves in similar circumstances. I want to empower you to take control of your health by making informed choices that support your body's natural healing processes. The principles of an alkaline diet can help create an environment in which cancer cells struggle to thrive, and my hope is that you, too, can experience the benefits of this lifestyle.

Throughout the chapters, you will find practical advice, personal anecdotes, and research-backed insights into how an alkaline diet can play a pivotal role in fighting cancer. From understanding the science behind pH levels to crafting meal plans and recipes that nourish your body, this book aims to provide you with the tools and knowledge you need to embark on your own journey toward healing.

You will learn not only about the foods to embrace and those to avoid but also about the broader lifestyle changes that can enhance your overall well-being. Mindset, community support, and stress management are all crucial components of this fight, and I will guide you through each aspect.

As you turn the pages, I invite you to reflect on your own journey and consider the possibilities that lie ahead. Together, we can explore the potential of natural healing, and I hope you will emerge empowered, inspired, and ready to take the next steps in your fight against cancer. Your path to wellness starts here.

1 My Journey to Fighting Cancer with an Alkaline Diet

Receiving a cancer diagnosis can feel like a seismic shock, shaking the very foundation of your life. When I first heard the words "you have cancer," I was engulfed by a whirlwind of emotions: disbelief, fear, and an overwhelming sense of vulnerability. The reality of my diagnosis hit me like a freight train, and suddenly, my future felt uncertain and precarious.

In those initial days, I struggled to process the news.

Questions flooded my mind:

"How could this be happening to me?" That was my first thought. I had always made wise decisions regarding my health. When I was diagnosed with cervical cancer, a type that I was told is one of the slowest-growing, I was devastated. My doctor made it clear: "There's nothing you can do." I was left feeling powerless, and I panicked, assuming I would eventually succumb to it. Yet, ten years later, I was still alive—and cancer-free—and I couldn't understand why.

I had never received any conventional treatment for cancer—no chemotherapy, no radiation, no surgeries. So, what had kept me alive and thriving? The answer was simpler than I could have imagined: I changed my diet. Specifically, I transitioned to an alkaline diet, a decision that came after six or seven years of living with untreated cancer.

I first heard about the benefits of an alkaline diet from a wealthy man I met in Miami who had knowledge about cancer from his own experience. He explained to me that cancer cells struggle to survive in an alkaline environment, but he only recommended drinking alkaline water. While I was already vegetarian and mostly vegan in my efforts to beat cancer, this conversation pushed me to take a further step— integrating more alkaline foods and water into my life.

I started by drinking alkaline water, which has a higher pH level than regular tap water. In the midst of this chaos, I found solace in research. I read medical journals and articles about alternative treatments in cancer. It was during this exploration that I stumbled upon the concept of an alkaline diet. Intrigued by the idea that the foods we consume can influence our body's pH levels and potentially impact cancer growth, I felt a glimmer of hope. This wasn't just about following another diet; it was about taking an active role in my health and well-being.

I began to learn about the principles of an alkaline diet— emphasizing fruits, vegetables, nuts, and seeds while minimizing processed foods, sugar, and animal products. The science behind it fascinated me: an alkaline environment in the body can create conditions less favorable for cancer cells, which thrive in acidity. I felt compelled to give this approach a try, believing it could serve as a complementary tool in my fight against cancer.

I also began focusing on foods that were known for their alkalizing effects, such as lemons, leafy greens, and vegetables like collards, spinach and kale. At the same time, I reduced my intake of acidic foods, like certain beans, which I found challenging since they had been my primary source of protein and iron as a vegetarian.

Over time, I noticed changes not only in my physical health but also in my mental clarity and energy levels. I began to see food not just as sustenance but as a source of healing. I discovered how to create meals that were vibrant, satisfying, and nourishing. I also noticed that eating healthy meant that I ate less and felt more nourished and satiated throughout the day. After consuming my daily iron, typically through black beans, I was able to walk 9 miles a day consistently.

Fast forward to a pelvic MRI I had after an unrelated accident, and I was in for the shock of my life: I was cancer-free. Not only that, but I was also free of HPV. I hadn't expected it, but my diet, combined with exercise and healthier lifestyle choices, had worked. I was ecstatic, overjoyed, and most of all—relieved.

I can't say this approach will work for everyone, especially for those with more aggressive or multiple tumors. There are certainly cases in which chemotherapy, radiation, or other treatments may be required. However, I'm convinced that the shift to an alkaline diet played a key role in reducing my cancer growth and accelerating my healing.

When I began to research the science behind it, I discovered that there is growing evidence to support the idea that diet can influence the body's pH balance and, in turn, affect cancer growth. Some studies suggest that cancer cells may thrive in more acidic environments, and while more research is needed, it's clear that nutrition plays a major role in overall health and disease prevention.

That's why I want to share this approach with you. I firmly believe in the power of nutrition and the benefits of focusing on alkaline foods. Now, I feel healthier and more energetic than ever before, and I owe much of that to the changes I made in my diet.

2 Understanding Cancer

Cancer can arise in nearly any organ or tissue and is classified into various types based on the nature of the cells involved and their location of origin. Understanding cancer is essential for anyone facing a diagnosis, as it lays the groundwork for exploring treatment options, including alternative approaches like an alkaline diet.

Cancer is a complex and often misunderstood disease that can take many forms. It arises from the uncontrolled growth of abnormal cells in the body, which can invade surrounding tissues and spread to other parts of the body. Understanding cancer requires a look at the underlying biological processes that fuel its development, as well as the risk factors that contribute to its progression. In this chapter, we will explore how cancer develops, the key risk factors associated with the disease, and the critical role that inflammation and acidity play in its growth.

The Development of Cancer: A Breakdown of Cellular Chaos

At its core, cancer is a result of cells behaving abnormally. Normally, the cells in our bodies grow, divide, and die in a controlled manner. Healthy cells follow instructions given by their DNA, ensuring that when they divide, they produce exact copies of themselves, maintaining balance in the body. This balance is essential for tissue repair, immune defense, and overall health.

However, when a cell's DNA is damaged or altered in a way that interferes with these natural instructions, it can begin to grow and divide uncontrollably. These abnormal cells don't die when they should, and instead, they continue to multiply, forming a mass known as a tumor. Tumors can be benign (non-cancerous) or malignant (cancerous). Malignant tumors have the dangerous ability to invade nearby tissues and organs and, through the bloodstream or lymphatic system, metastasize to other areas of the body, making the disease more difficult to treat.

The development of cancer is often a slow process, occurring over many years as mutations accumulate in the DNA. These mutations can be triggered by a variety of factors, including genetics, environmental influences, and lifestyle choices.

Risk Factors: What Increases the Chances of Cancer?

Cancer is a multifaceted disease with numerous risk factors. Some are unavoidable, while others are modifiable, giving individuals the power to reduce their risk. The most common risk factors include:

- **Genetics**: Family history plays a significant role in determining cancer risk. Certain genetic mutations are inherited and can predispose individuals to specific types of cancer. For example, mutations in the BRCA1 and BRCA2 genes are linked to higher rates of breast and ovarian cancer.

- **Environmental Exposure**: Harmful substances in the environment, such as radiation, toxic chemicals, and pollutants, can damage DNA and increase cancer risk. Prolonged exposure to UV rays from the sun can lead to skin cancer, while exposure to carcinogenic chemicals like asbestos or smoke can cause lung and other forms of cancer.

- **Lifestyle Choices**: Lifestyle factors like smoking, excessive alcohol consumption, poor diet, and lack of physical activity are known contributors to cancer development. Smoking is one of the leading causes of lung cancer, while a diet high in processed foods and sugar is associated with various types of cancer, including colorectal cancer.

- **Chronic Inflammation**: Ongoing inflammation in the body, often caused by infection, autoimmune disorders, or obesity, can increase the risk of cancer. Inflammation triggers cellular changes and DNA damage, making it easier for abnormal cells to grow.

- **Acidity and Diet**: As we'll explore in more detail, an acidic internal environment caused by a poor diet, stress, and lack of oxygen can promote the conditions cancer cells thrive in.

The Biological Processes of Cancer

Cancer isn't just one disease—it's a collection of over 100 different diseases, each with its own unique characteristics. However, all forms of cancer share some common traits. These include:

1. **Uncontrolled Cell Division**: Cancer cells bypass the normal regulatory mechanisms that control cell growth and division. They continue to multiply even when the body doesn't need more cells, leading to tumor formation.

2. **Invasion and Metastasis**: Unlike healthy cells, cancer cells can invade nearby tissues and organs. In advanced stages, cancer cells break away from the original tumor and travel through the bloodstream or lymphatic system, forming new tumors in distant locations. This is known as metastasis.

3. **Evading Immune Surveillance**: The immune system's role is to identify and destroy abnormal or damaged cells, including cancer cells. However, cancer cells have developed ways to evade immune detection, allowing them to grow unchecked.

4. **Sustaining Inflammation**: Many cancers thrive in inflammatory environments. Chronic inflammation promotes the release of growth

factors that fuel cancer cell proliferation, aiding in their ability to invade tissues and spread.

The Role of Inflammation and Acidity in Cancer Progression

While cancer has many causes, two of the most important factors in its progression are chronic inflammation and acidity. Both play significant roles in creating an internal environment that is conducive to the growth and spread of cancer.

Inflammation and Cancer

Inflammation is the body's natural response to injury or infection. In short-term scenarios, it's a helpful process that promotes healing. However, when inflammation becomes chronic, it can cause extensive damage to tissues and DNA, laying the groundwork for cancer development. Chronic inflammatory conditions, such as Crohn's disease, ulcerative colitis, and hepatitis, are known to increase cancer risk because the constant irritation and cellular turnover promote abnormal cell growth.

Inflammation also provides cancer cells with the tools they need to thrive. The inflammatory process releases cytokines and other chemicals that promote cellular proliferation, aid in tumor blood vessel formation (angiogenesis), and enable cancer cells to evade immune detection.

Acidity: Fertile Ground for Cancer Growth

Just as plants thrive in specific soil conditions, cancer cells thrive in a specific internal environment—one that is acidic and low in oxygen. Acidity and cancer progression are tightly linked. When the body becomes too acidic due to poor diet, stress, and lack of oxygen, it creates an environment that cancer cells can easily exploit.

In an acidic state, cells are deprived of sufficient oxygen, which forces them to switch from aerobic (oxygen-based) metabolism to anaerobic (non-oxygen-based) metabolism. Cancer cells prefer anaerobic conditions because it allows them to grow and multiply rapidly. Unlike healthy cells, which require oxygen to function properly, cancer cells are remarkably adaptable to acidic, oxygen-poor environments, making them difficult to eliminate.

This acidic environment also weakens the immune system's ability to fight off cancer cells. A body in acidosis has a harder time identifying and destroying abnormal cells, allowing them to grow unchecked. That's why promoting a more alkaline internal state through diet and lifestyle changes is crucial in cancer prevention and treatment.

Overview of Cancer Types and Stages

Cancer is categorized into several major groups:

1. **Carcinomas**: These cancers originate from epithelial cells that line the surfaces of organs and tissues. They are the most common type and include:

   - **Breast cancer**

   - **Lung cancer**

   - **Colorectal cancer**

   - **Prostate cancer**

2. **Sarcomas**: These tumors arise from connective tissues, such as bones, muscles, and cartilage. While less common, they can be aggressive. Examples include:

   - **Osteosarcoma** (bone cancer)

   - **Liposarcoma** (fat tissue cancer)

3. **Leukemias**: Cancers of the blood and bone marrow, leukemias result in the production of abnormal blood cells. Key types include:

   - **Acute myeloid leukemia (AML)**

   - **Chronic lymphocytic leukemia (CLL)**

4. **Lymphomas**: These cancers begin in the lymphatic system and include:

   - **Hodgkin lymphoma**

   - **Non-Hodgkin lymphoma**

5. **Central Nervous System (CNS) Cancers**:
    These tumors affect the brain and spinal cord,
    presenting unique challenges and treatment
    considerations.

Staging of Cancer

Once diagnosed, cancer is staged to determine its extent
and severity. Staging helps guide treatment decisions and
predict outcomes. The most common staging system
includes:

- **Stage I**: The cancer is localized, small, and has
  not spread.

- **Stage II**: The tumor is larger but still localized,
  with possible involvement of nearby lymph
  nodes.

- **Stage III**: The cancer has spread to nearby lymph
  nodes and possibly surrounding tissues.

- **Stage IV**: The cancer has metastasized,
  spreading to distant parts of the body.

This classification is crucial for understanding treatment
options and prognosis.

Explanation of Conventional Treatments

Conventional cancer treatments aim to eliminate cancer
cells while minimizing damage to healthy tissues. The
main modalities include:

1. **Surgery**: Often the first line of treatment for localized tumors, surgery involves the removal of the tumor and surrounding tissue. It can also include biopsies to determine the cancer type and stage. Surgical intervention may provide the best chance for a cure, particularly if the cancer is detected early.

2. **Chemotherapy**: This systemic treatment uses powerful drugs to target and destroy rapidly dividing cancer cells. Chemotherapy can be administered intravenously or orally and is often used in conjunction with surgery and radiation. While effective, it may cause significant side effects, including nausea, hair loss, and fatigue, due to its impact on healthy cells.

3. **Radiation Therapy**: Utilizing high-energy radiation, this treatment aims to kill cancer cells or shrink tumors. It can be applied externally (from a machine) or internally (through implanted radioactive material). Radiation is commonly used before surgery to reduce tumor size or after surgery to eliminate residual cancer cells.

4. **Targeted Therapy**: These therapies focus on specific molecular targets associated with cancer cells, blocking their growth and spread while minimizing harm to normal cells. Targeted therapies have revolutionized cancer treatment

for certain types of cancer, offering more personalized approaches.

5. **Immunotherapy**: This innovative treatment harnesses the body's immune system to fight cancer. By enhancing the immune response or providing immune components, immunotherapy has shown promise in improving outcomes for various cancers.

While conventional treatments are often effective, they come with challenges, including side effects and varying rates of success. This understanding sets the stage for exploring complementary approaches, such as an alkaline diet, which may support overall health during cancer treatment.

pH and Cancer Connection

In this chapter, we've explored how cancer develops, the risk factors that contribute to its progression, and the biological processes that allow it to thrive. The role of inflammation and acidity cannot be overstated—both contribute significantly to the conditions that support cancer cell growth.

As we move forward, we will examine how adjusting your diet to promote an alkaline state can help reduce acidity and inflammation, thereby creating a less hospitable environment for cancer cells. Understanding the connection between pH balance and cancer is key to making informed choices for your long-term health and well-being.

3 Alkalinity and Its Role in Cancer Prevention

Cancer is one of the most feared diseases worldwide, but growing research suggests that we may have more control over preventing it than we think. One promising area of study focuses on the relationship between the body's pH balance and cancer. Specifically, how maintaining an alkaline environment through diet and lifestyle may help suppress cancer cell growth and reduce the risk of developing the disease.

In this chapter, we'll explore the scientific studies linking an alkaline environment to cancer suppression, the biological mechanisms behind this connection, and how an alkaline diet can help maintain optimal pH balance to prevent cancer cell proliferation.

The Science Behind Alkalinity and Cancer Suppression

Over the past few decades, researchers have studied the impact of pH balance on cellular health. The body functions best when its pH is slightly alkaline, typically around 7.35 to 7.45. This balance is critical for various biological processes, including cell metabolism, immune function, and the maintenance of a healthy internal environment.

However, modern lifestyles—characterized by stress, poor diet, lack of physical activity, and exposure to toxins—can tip the scales toward acidity. In an acidic environment, the body's cells, particularly cancer cells, can thrive. Studies have shown that cancer cells prefer a more acidic environment, while healthy cells function optimally in a slightly alkaline one.

Several scientific studies support the idea that alkalinity can play a significant role in cancer prevention:

1. **Otto Warburg's Hypothesis on Cancer Metabolism**
   Nobel Prize-winning biochemist Dr. Otto Warburg was one of the first to propose a link between acidity and cancer. His groundbreaking research demonstrated that cancer cells generate energy primarily through a process called anaerobic glycolysis, even in the presence of oxygen. This process allows cancer cells to survive and proliferate in acidic environments by using glucose for energy. Warburg suggested that cancer cells could be suppressed in an alkaline, oxygen-rich environment, as they would be less able to sustain their rapid growth.

2. **Research on pH and Tumor Growth**
   More recent studies have built on Warburg's work. In 2009, a study published in the journal *Cancer Research* examined the effects of acidic and alkaline conditions on tumor growth. The researchers found that an acidic microenvironment promoted tumor invasion, while an alkaline microenvironment hindered it.

By neutralizing the acidity around cancer cells, researchers were able to reduce tumor growth, providing further evidence that pH plays a vital role in cancer progression.

3. **Alkaline Diet and Its Anti-Cancer Potential**
   Research also suggests that diet can influence the body's pH levels, and an alkaline diet may offer protection against cancer. A study published in *The British Journal of Nutrition* found that an alkaline diet rich in fruits, vegetables, and plant-based foods can create an internal environment less conducive to cancer cell growth. This diet minimizes the intake of acid-forming foods like processed meats, refined sugars, and alcohol, which are known to promote an acidic environment.

These studies highlight the potential for alkalinity to suppress cancer by inhibiting its ability to grow in an acidic environment. They also suggest that making dietary and lifestyle changes to support pH balance can be a powerful tool in cancer prevention.

How an Alkaline Diet Maintains pH Balance

An alkaline diet is not just about what you eat; it's about promoting an overall lifestyle that fosters balance in the body. The foods we consume have either an alkalizing or acidifying effect once metabolized. By understanding how different foods influence the body's pH, you can make informed choices that support long-term health and cancer prevention.

Alkaline-Forming Foods
Alkaline-forming foods are those that help neutralize excess acidity in the body and promote a slightly alkaline pH. These foods are generally plant-based and packed with nutrients that support cellular health and immune function. Some of the most alkalizing foods include:

- Leafy greens like collards, spinach, kale, and Swiss chard

- Cruciferous vegetables such as broccoli, cauliflower, and Brussels sprouts

- Fruits like lemons, limes, avocados, and berries (even though citrus fruits are acidic before digestion, they have an alkalizing effect in the body)

- Root vegetables such as sweet potatoes, beets, and carrots

- Nuts and seeds, particularly pumpkin seeds, almonds and flaxseeds

- Legumes and beans like lentils, chickpeas, and black beans

- Herbal teas and green tea

These foods provide essential minerals like magnesium, potassium, and calcium, which act as natural buffers to counteract acidity. Additionally, their high fiber content helps maintain a healthy gut, which is crucial for balancing pH and reducing inflammation—a key factor in cancer prevention.

Acid-Forming Foods to Avoid

On the flip side, certain foods can contribute to acidity and create an internal environment more favorable to cancer cell growth. These acid-forming foods are often highly processed, refined, and laden with chemicals. Some of the most acidifying foods include:

- Processed meats (bacon, sausage, hot dogs)

- Refined sugars and sugary beverages

- Dairy products like cheese and whole milk

- White bread and pasta made from refined grains

- Alcohol

- Caffeine, especially from sugary energy drinks

- Fried and fast foods

- Artificial sweeteners and additives

While it's impossible to avoid all acid-forming foods, reducing their intake and emphasizing alkaline-forming foods can significantly help maintain a balanced pH.

Preventing Cancer Cell Proliferation Through Diet
Cancer cells thrive in acidic, oxygen-deprived environments, but they struggle to survive in alkaline conditions. By adopting an alkaline diet, you can help create an environment that reduces the likelihood of cancer cell proliferation.

Oxygen and Cellular Health
When the body's pH leans toward alkalinity, cells receive more oxygen, which is essential for healthy cellular function. Cancer cells are anaerobic, meaning they generate energy without using oxygen, which allows them to survive and multiply in low-oxygen conditions. By improving oxygenation through alkalinity, you make it harder for cancer cells to thrive.

Reducing Inflammation
An alkaline diet also helps combat inflammation, which is a known precursor to many types of cancer. Chronic inflammation can damage cellular DNA, creating mutations that lead to cancer. Foods rich in antioxidants, vitamins, and minerals—like those found in an alkaline diet—help neutralize harmful free radicals and reduce inflammation, providing another layer of protection against cancer.

Improved Immune Function
A balanced pH strengthens the immune system, making it more efficient at detecting and destroying abnormal cells before they have a chance to develop into cancer. Alkaline-forming foods, particularly leafy greens and

fruits, are loaded with immune-boosting nutrients like vitamin C, zinc, and selenium. By supporting the body's natural defense mechanisms, you can lower your cancer risk and improve overall health.

Empowering Prevention Through pH Balance

Maintaining an alkaline internal environment through diet and lifestyle may be one of the most effective tools we have in the fight against cancer. Scientific studies show that alkalinity can suppress cancer cell growth by promoting oxygenation, reducing inflammation, and supporting immune function. By prioritizing alkaline-forming foods and minimizing acid-forming ones, you can create a body that is less hospitable to cancer cells and more equipped to prevent disease.

4 The Science Behind the Alkaline Diet

The alkaline diet has garnered attention for its potential role in promoting health and preventing disease, particularly cancer. At the core of this dietary approach is the concept of pH levels and the body's natural balance. Understanding these principles can shed light on how an alkaline diet may influence cancer cell behavior.

Explanation of pH Levels and the Body's Natural Balance

pH Levels: The pH scale measures how acidic or alkaline a substance is, ranging from 0 (very acidic) to 14 (very alkaline), with 7 being neutral. As I've already mentioned, the human body operates best at a slightly alkaline pH level, around 7.4. Maintaining this balance is crucial for optimal physiological function.

Acid-Base Balance: The body regulates its pH through various mechanisms, including respiration, metabolism, and renal function. When the body becomes too acidic (a condition known as acidosis), it can disrupt metabolic processes and potentially lead to health issues. Chronic acidosis has been linked to a variety of diseases, including cancer.

Buffering Systems: The body employs buffering systems to neutralize excess acids. Bicarbonate ions, proteins, and phosphate play vital roles in maintaining pH balance. However, when these systems are overwhelmed—often due to poor dietary choices—the body may struggle to maintain an optimal pH level.

The Alkaline Environment and Immune Function

At the core of the alkaline diet is the belief that dietary choices can influence the body's pH levels. While the body naturally regulates its pH, certain foods can create a more alkaline environment, which proponents argue may enhance immune function.

Cellular Mechanisms

When the body is in a more alkaline state, several cellular processes can be positively affected:

1. **Oxygen Availability**: Cancer cells thrive in acidic environments, where oxygen levels are often lower. Alkaline diets, rich in fruits and vegetables, are high in antioxidants and vitamins that enhance oxygen transport in the blood. Increased oxygen availability may inhibit cancer cell proliferation, as most cancerous cells rely on anaerobic respiration.

2. **Reduced Inflammation**: Chronic inflammation is a significant contributor to cancer development. An alkaline diet is associated with lower levels of inflammation in the body. Foods like leafy greens, nuts, and seeds contain anti-inflammatory compounds that can modulate immune responses, potentially decreasing the risk of cancer.

3. **Enhanced Immune Response**: An alkaline environment can promote the activity of immune cells, such as T-cells and natural killer cells, which are crucial for detecting and destroying cancer cells. Research suggests that a diet high in alkaline foods may lead to an increase in these immune cell populations, enhancing the body's ability to fight off tumors.

Impact of Alkaline Foods on Cancer Markers

Several studies have investigated the effects of alkaline foods on specific cancer markers. These markers are substances in the body that indicate the presence or progression of cancer.

Key Findings

1. **Decreased Tumor Markers**: A study published in the *Journal of Clinical Oncology* indicated that patients who adopted a predominantly alkaline diet showed reduced levels of certain tumor markers, such as prostate-specific antigen (PSA) and cancer antigen 125 (CA-125). This suggests a potential link between dietary pH and cancer progression.

2. **Cellular Regeneration**: Alkaline foods, particularly those rich in vitamins C and E, have been shown to enhance cellular regeneration. This is crucial for recovering from treatments like chemotherapy, where normal cells can also

be damaged. Nutrient-dense, alkaline foods support the repair processes within the cells, promoting healthier cell turnover.

3. **Antioxidant Activity**: Foods commonly included in an alkaline diet, such as berries, citrus fruits, and cruciferous vegetables, are rich in antioxidants. These compounds combat oxidative stress, a significant factor in cancer development. By neutralizing free radicals, alkaline foods may help prevent cellular damage that can lead to malignancy.

The alkaline diet posits that creating a more alkaline internal environment can strengthen immune function and potentially reduce cancer risk. While further research is needed to establish definitive causal relationships, existing studies suggest that an alkaline diet may positively influence cancer markers and promote cellular regeneration. As we continue to explore the interplay between diet and health, understanding these cellular mechanisms offers promising avenues for enhancing cancer prevention strategies and supporting overall well-being.

5 Key Principles of an Alkaline Diet

Adopting an alkaline diet involves understanding which foods support an alkaline environment in the body and which ones contribute to acidity. This chapter will outline the key principles cf an alkaline diet, focusing on foods to embrace and those to avoid.

Before we begin, it's important to grasp the concepts of alkalinity and the pH scale. The pH scale measures how acidic or alkaline a substance is, ranging from 0 to 14. A pH of 0 indicates the highest acidity, while 14 represents the highest alkalinity. A value of 7 is the neutral state.

Specifically, pH reflects the concentration of free hydrogen and hydroxyl ions in a solution. If a substance contains more hydroxyl ions than hydrogen ions, it is considered basic or alkaline. Conversely, if there are more hydrogen ions than hydroxyl ions, the substance is deemed acidic.

When selecting foods to include in your diet, aim for options with a pH of 7 or higher. Throughout my journey, I focused on foods with a pH of 8 or above and completely avoided any mildly acidic options.

Below is a list of the foods I chose. Following that, we'll look at other foods that are safe to incorporate if you prefer a different approach.

High and Low Alkaline Foods

It's important to note that certain foods have higher alkalinity when consumed fresh, such as cherries, while others, like oats, become more alkaline when cooked. Additionally, some foods may exhibit a more alkaline effect in the body than their pH levels would suggest when tested outside the body.

Mixed Greens (Collards, Spinach, Kale)

- **Rich in Nutrients:** High in vitamins A, C, K, and various B vitamins, mixed greens are excellent for immune support and skin health.

- **Antioxidant Properties:** They contain antioxidants that combat oxidative stress, reducing the risk of chronic diseases.

- **Digestive Health:** Their fiber content promotes healthy digestion and may help in maintaining a healthy weight.

Seaweed

- **Nutrient-Rich**: Packed with vitamins (A, C, E, K, and B vitamins) and minerals (iodine, calcium, iron, magnesium).

- **High in Fiber**: Supports digestion, promotes gut health, and aids in weight management.

- **Antioxidant and Anti-inflammatory**: Contains compounds that combat oxidative stress and inflammation, potentially reducing the risk of chronic diseases.

Cucumbers

- **Hydration:** Composed of about 95% water, cucumbers help keep you hydrated.

- **Low in Calories:** A low-calorie food that can help with weight management.

- **Anti-inflammatory Properties:** Contains anti-inflammatory compounds that may benefit skin health.

Carrots

- **Vision Health:** Rich in beta-carotene, which converts to vitamin A, carrots support good vision.

- **High in Fiber:** Promotes digestive health and may help lower cholesterol levels.

- **Antioxidant Effects:** Contains antioxidants that help fight free radicals in the body.

Avocados

- **Healthy Fats:** Rich in monounsaturated fats, avocados support heart health and help regulate cholesterol levels.

- **Nutrient Dense:** Packed with vitamins, minerals, and fiber, contributing to overall health.

- **Anti-inflammatory Properties:** May help reduce inflammation and promote skin health.

Purple Cabbage

- **High in Antioxidants:** Contains anthocyanins, which have been linked to reduced risk of chronic diseases.

- **Digestive Health:** Fiber-rich, purple cabbage promotes a healthy digestive system.

- **Supports Immune Function:** Rich in vitamins C and K, which are crucial for immune health.

Sweet Potatoes

- **Rich in Beta-Carotene:** Provides antioxidants that support eye health and may reduce cancer risk.

- **Blood Sugar Regulation:** High fiber content helps regulate blood sugar levels.

- **Nutrient Dense:** Packed with vitamins A, C, and potassium, beneficial for heart health.

Red Grapes, Cherries

- **Rich in Antioxidants:** Contain resveratrol and other polyphenols that may support heart health and reduce inflammation.

- **Anti-inflammatory Effects:** Cherries can help reduce muscle soreness and inflammation.

- **Support Sleep:** Cherries are a natural source of melatonin, which can improve sleep quality, but are most effective when consumed fresh.

Lemons, Limes

- **Vitamin C Boost:** High in vitamin C, supporting immune function and skin health.

- **Digestive Aid:** May help improve digestion and detoxification when consumed in water.

- **Alkalizing Effect:** Despite their acidity, they have an alkalizing effect on the body after digestion.

Bell Peppers

- **High in Vitamins:** Particularly rich in vitamins A and C, bell peppers support immune function and skin health.

- **Antioxidant Properties:** Contain various antioxidants that protect against oxidative stress.

- **Weight Management:** Low in calories and high in fiber, they promote satiety.

Beets

- **Detoxification Support:** Beets help support liver function and detoxification.

- **Rich in Folate:** Important for DNA synthesis and repair, crucial for overall health.

- **Improved Athletic Performance:** May enhance stamina due to nitrates, which improve blood flow.

Red Onions, Garlic

- **Heart Health:** Both contain compounds that can help lower cholesterol and blood pressure.

- **Antimicrobial Properties:** Garlic has well-documented antimicrobial and anti-inflammatory properties.

- **Rich in Antioxidants:** They help protect against cellular damage and support immune health.

Zucchini

- **Low in Calories:** A low-calorie food that can aid in weight management.

- **Hydrating Properties:** High water content helps with hydration.

- **Rich in Nutrients:** Contains vitamins A and C, promoting overall health.

White Navy Beans

- **High in Protein and Fiber:** Support muscle health and digestive function.

- **Nutrient Dense:** A good source of vitamins and minerals, including iron and magnesium.

- **Blood Sugar Regulation:** Their high fiber content helps stabilize blood sugar levels.

Ginger, Basil

- **Anti-inflammatory Effects:** Both have properties that may help reduce inflammation and pain.

- **Digestive Health:** Ginger is particularly well-known for aiding digestion and reducing nausea.

- **Antioxidant Properties:** Both herbs provide antioxidants that support overall health.

Chia Seeds, Flax Seeds

- **Omega-3 Fatty Acids:** Rich in plant-based omega-3s, beneficial for heart health.

- **High in Fiber:** Promote digestive health and may aid in weight management.

- **Nutrient Dense:** Provide protein, vitamins, and minerals, contributing to overall nutrition.

Himalayan Sea Salt

- **Electrolyte Balance:** Provides essential minerals that help maintain electrolyte balance.

- **Flavor Enhancer:** Can enhance the flavor of foods without the need for processed salts.

- **Alkalizing Properties:** May help maintain pH balance in the body.

Lentils

- **High in Protein and Fiber:** Support muscle growth and digestive health.

- **Nutrient Dense:** Rich in iron, folate, and various vitamins and minerals.

- **Blood Sugar Control:** Their high fiber content helps regulate blood sugar levels.

Artichokes, Asparagus

- **Digestive Health:** Both are high in fiber, promoting a healthy digestive system.

- **Antioxidant Properties:** Contain antioxidants that may help protect against chronic diseases.

- **Support Liver Health:** Artichokes are particularly known for their liver-supporting properties.

Incorporating these alkaline foods into your diet can enhance overall health, support cancer prevention, and contribute to a balanced and nutritious lifestyle.

Here are the nutritional benefits of mildly acidic foods:

Black Beans, Chickpeas

- **Nutritional Benefits:**

- o **High in Protein:** Excellent plant-based protein sources, supporting muscle health.

- o **Rich in Fiber:** Promotes digestive health and helps regulate blood sugar levels.

- o **Nutrient Dense:** Contains vitamins and minerals such as iron, magnesium, and folate, essential for overall health.

Cantaloupe, Watermelon

- **Nutritional Benefits:**

  - o **Hydration:** High water content helps keep you hydrated.

  - o **Vitamins A and C:** Supports immune function, skin health, and vision.

  - o **Low in Calories:** A healthy snack option that aids in weight management.

Blackberries, Blueberries

- **Nutritional Benefits:**

  - o **High in Antioxidants:** Rich in vitamins C and K, and anthocyanins that protect against oxidative stress.

  - o **Anti-Inflammatory:** May reduce inflammation and support heart health.

o   **Fiber Content:** Supports digestive health and helps maintain a healthy weight.

Pineapples, Strawberries

- **Nutritional Benefits:**

  o   **Vitamin C Boost:** Both fruits are high in vitamin C, enhancing immune function and skin health.

  o   **Digestive Health:** Pineapples contain bromelain, which aids digestion; strawberries are high in fiber.

  o   **Hydration:** Both fruits have high water content, promoting hydration.

Oats, Wild Rice

- **Nutritional Benefits:**

  o   **Whole Grains:** Rich in fiber, which supports digestive health and helps control blood sugar levels.

  o   **Nutrient Dense:** Contains essential vitamins and minerals such as B vitamins, iron, and magnesium.

  o   **Heart Health:** Oats are known for their cholesterol-lowering properties.

Cranberries

- **Nutritional Benefits:**

Although cranberries are acidic with a pH range between 2.3 and 2.5, they possess strong antibacterial properties. Fresh cranberries are less acidic than cranberry juice, dried cranberries, and cooked cranberries and have a more alkalizing effect in the body, making them the preferred option.

- **High in Antioxidants:** Rich in vitamins C and E, helping combat oxidative stress.

- **Urinary Health:** Though acidic, may help prevent urinary tract infections due to their proanthocyanidin content.

- **Anti-Inflammatory:** Supports overall health and may reduce inflammation in the body.

Incorporating these mildly acidic foods into your diet can provide various health benefits, contributing to overall well-being and nutritional balance.

Here are reasons to avoid these acidic foods:

Refined Sugar, Alcohol

- **Impact on pH Balance:** Can lead to increased acidity in the body, promoting an unfavorable environment for health.

- Nutrient Deficiency: High in calories but low in nutrients, contributing to weight gain and potential health issues.

- Inflammation: Both can promote inflammation, leading to chronic health problems.

Cocoa, Dried Fruit

- **High Sugar Content:** Many dried fruits contain added sugars, increasing acidity and calorie content.

- **Potential for Weight Gain:** Overconsumption can lead to weight gain and associated health risks.

- **Acidic Nature**: Cocoa can be acidic, which may contribute to digestive issues for some individuals.

Vinegar, Miso, Soy Sauce

- **High Sodium Content:** Can contribute to high blood pressure and other cardiovascular issues.

- **Acidic pH:** May disrupt the body's pH balance and lead to digestive discomfort.

- **Fermented Products:** While they have some benefits, they can be acidic and exacerbate conditions like acid reflux.

White Rice

- **Low Nutritional Value:** Lacks fiber and essential nutrients compared to whole grains.

- **High Glycemic Index**: Can cause spikes in blood sugar levels, leading to energy crashes and cravings.

- **Acidic Impact:** Can contribute to overall acidity in the diet.

Mushrooms

- **Acidic Nature:** Certain mushrooms can be acidic, potentially affecting pH balance.

- **Allergenic Potential:** Some people may have sensitivities or allergies to specific types of mushrooms.

- **Digestive Issues:** Can cause bloating or discomfort in sensitive individuals.

Bread, Yeast

- **Gluten Content:** Can be inflammatory for those with gluten sensitivities or celiac disease.

- **High in Refined Carbs:** May lead to blood sugar spikes and subsequent crashes.

- **Acidic Nature:** Fermentation processes can lead to acidity in the body.

Honey, Jelly, Rice Syrup

- **High Sugar Levels:** Can lead to increased acidity and weight gain, like refined sugars.

- **Caloric Density:** Low in nutritional value while being high in calories.

- **Inflammation:** Can promote inflammation in the body when consumed excessively.

Soda, Carbonated Water

- **High Sugar and Acidity:** Regular sodas are high in sugar and can contribute to acid buildup in the body.

- **Bone Health:** Can lead to lower bone density due to increased acidity.

- **Dental Health Risks:** High acidity can erode tooth enamel.

Ketchup, Mustard

- **Added Sugars and Preservatives:** Often contain sugars and additives that can affect health negatively.

- **Acidic Ingredients:** High acidity can lead to digestive issues for some individuals.

- **Low Nutritional Value:** Generally low in essential nutrients.

Eggs, Shellfish, Meat

- **Acidic Nature:** High protein foods can increase acidity in the body.

- **Saturated Fats:** Some meats and shellfish are high in saturated fats, which can impact heart health.

- **Environmental Concerns:** High consumption may contribute to environmental issues related to livestock farming.

Snack Foods (Chips, Cookies, and Popcorn)

- **Refined Carbohydrates:** These foods are often made from refined flours and sugars, contributing to higher acidity in the body.
- **Low Nutritional Value:** Typically, low in essential nutrients like vitamins and minerals, they offer little health benefit while increasing acid load.
- **Processed Oils and Additives:** Chips and cookies often contain unhealthy fats and preservatives, which can promote inflammation and are linked to cancer progression.

Avoiding these acidic foods can help maintain a healthier pH balance in the body, support overall well-being, and reduce the risk of chronic health conditions.

Other Foods to Embrace

1. **Vegetables:**
   - **Alkaline Benefits**: Vegetables are a cornerstone of the alkaline diet, providing essential nutrients and fiber while helping to maintain pH balance.
   - **Examples**:
     - **Cruciferous Vegetables**: Broccoli, cauliflower, and Brussels sprouts support detoxification and are rich in cancer-fighting compounds.
     - **Root Vegetables**: Beets and carrots offer vitamins and minerals while promoting alkalinity.

2. **Nuts and Seeds**:
   - **Alkaline Benefits**: Nuts and seeds are excellent sources of healthy fats, protein, and essential nutrients, promoting overall health. Keep in mind that certain nuts and seeds are more acidic than others. In general, peanuts should be avoided if battling cancer. Since I have a nut and seed (most except flax seeds, sesame seeds, and pumpkin seeds) allergy, this was easy for me to avoid.
   - **Examples**:

- **Chia Seeds**: Packed with omega-3 fatty acids and fiber, chia seeds can help balance blood sugar and promote digestive health.

- **Flax seeds**: High in omega-3 fatty acids and rich in fiber. Flax Seeds may help stabilize blood sugar levels.

- **Pumpkin Seeds**: Rich in zinc and magnesium, pumpkin seeds also support immune function.

- **Almonds**: High in magnesium and vitamin E, almonds are a great alkaline snack.

3. **Whole Grains**:

   - **Alkaline Benefits**: Whole grains provide fiber and nutrients that can help maintain stable blood sugar levels and support digestive health.

   - **Examples**:

     - **Quinoa**: Quinoa is slightly acidic with a pH of 6.0 to 6.8, it is alkaline forming in the body. Although quinoa is gluten-free, I am allergic to quinoa, and thus, I cannot consume it.

- **Brown Rice**: Provides fiber and essential nutrients while being less acidic than white rice.

- **Oats**: Oats are in the pH range of A nutritious breakfast option that can be easily incorporated into an alkaline diet.

By focusing on embracing alkaline-promoting foods like fruits, vegetables, nuts, seeds, and whole grains, while avoiding processed foods, sugars, and animal products, individuals can significantly improve their overall health and potentially create an environment that is less hospitable to cancer.

Understanding Your Body

While eating alkaline foods is crucial, it's not as simple as just following a diet. Everyone's body is different, and it's important to know how your body reacts to specific foods. I recommend keeping a food journal as you transition to a new diet. Start with a brief fast, then slowly reintroduce foods one by one, paying close attention to how you feel.

For instance, while spinach is generally considered an excellent alkaline food, I personally cannot eat it due to my arthritis. Spinach contains lectins and oxalates, compounds that exacerbate my joint pain. However, someone without arthritis might consume it with no issues. This is why it's important to be mindful of your body's unique needs.

Consult with a holistic doctor or nutritionist to develop a cancer-fighting diet that won't worsen any existing health conditions. Ultimately, nutrition can play a powerful role in supporting your body, and when combined with other healthy practices, it can aid in healing.

I can't say enough about the importance of finding a diet that works for you. What I can say is that for me, an alkaline diet played a vital role in my recovery. While more research is needed on this subject, it's clear that the right nutrition can have a profound effect on our health.

In the following pages, I would like to discuss some health concerns that I had during my battle with cancer. Perhaps, some of my health concerns, can help others identify their own unique health problems and start you on your journey to developing a personalized alkaline diet that will provide optimal results for you.

During my battle with cancer, anemia became a significant challenge, and even now, I continue to struggle with it. My intestinal lining was damaged after prolonged exposure to untreated food allergens, impairing my ability to absorb and store iron properly. I once consumed so much iron daily that I nearly overdosed. So, I had to learn how to balance my iron levels carefully. However, I still must meet my daily iron requirements to avoid negative side effects.

My primary sources of iron, both then and now, include:

1. Lentils

2. Black beans

3. Chia seeds

4. Beets

5. Collards

These plant-based sources of iron have been the most sustainable for me. I found lentils and collards to be especially effective in managing my iron deficiency. On days when I consume them, I don't experience the intense hunger that plagued me when I neglected iron-rich foods.

For example, today I didn't have my usual cup of black beans. All day long, I had a nagging hunger headache, even after eating chickpeas, pumpkin seeds, mixed greens, avocado, and an entire loaf of gluten-free bread. Nothing could satisfy my hunger. On days when I eat my iron-rich foods, I often forget to eat more than one meal, as iron helps curb my appetite.

Before switching to a quasi-vegan diet, I assumed my constant hunger was due to a lack of protein. I would eat chicken for breakfast, lunch, and dinner, snack on peanuts, cashews, or almonds, and still feel unsatisfied.

It wasn't until I addressed my iron deficiency that I realized protein wasn't the issue—it was my need for plant-based iron. Once I incorporated more iron into my diet, I no longer felt the urge to consume excessive amounts of food, like eating three-quarters of a chicken every day.

However, while iron is essential for combating anemia and regulating weight, it can be detrimental in the fight against cancer. According to the National Institutes of Health (NIH):

"Elemental iron is essential for cellular growth and homeostasis, but it is potentially toxic to cells and tissues. High intake of dietary iron is associated with an increased risk for some cancers, particularly colorectal cancer."

Similarly, the New York Times has reported that:

"Menstruating women are unlikely to have a problem, but for others with high iron stores, recommended treatments include phlebotomy and frequent blood donation. Without these measures, excess iron can be deposited in the liver, heart, and pancreas, leading to cirrhosis, liver cancer, cardiac arrhythmias, and diabetes."

This makes it crucial to monitor iron levels, particularly during cancer treatment, to ensure that excess iron isn't contributing to the problem. Even with my diet of black beans, collards, and chia seeds, I still had low iron levels. When I came close to overdosing, it was because I had been taking a food-based vitamin that provided 100% of the recommended daily allowance of iron.

Most menstruating women don't need to worry about iron overload, but I always increase my iron intake before and during my period to prevent headaches and mental fog. Iron plays a critical role in brain function. Without sufficient iron, your body cannot produce enough red blood cells, which contain hemoglobin that carries oxygen to your brain. This can hinder both cognitive function, memory, and your body's ability to fight cancer.

According to WebMD, iron deficiencies can lead to memory loss. Fortunately, iron supplements can help reduce or reverse this memory impairment by increasing oxygen levels in the body.

Caveat Emptor:

As LiveStrong notes:

"Because blood loss usually accounts for low iron levels, certain cancers associated with bleeding—such as colon, rectal, stomach, and esophageal cancers—bring on anemia. Cancer thrives in an inflammatory state, and as it produces more inflammation, it causes body tissues to bleed."

Low iron not only creates a favorable environment for cancer but can also lead to other health issues like sensorineural hearing loss, heart palpitations, irritability, fatigue, and, of course, memory loss. Studies suggest that individuals with anemia are 2.4 times more likely to experience damage to blood vessels in the ear, leading to hearing loss. However, memory loss due to iron deficiency is usually temporary, provided iron levels are restored quickly.

Maintaining optimal iron levels is vital to a healthy lifestyle. While too little iron can contribute to anemia and exacerbate cancer, too much iron can be toxic and may increase the risk of certain cancers. Regular monitoring of iron levels is essential. Before making any dietary changes, consult with your physician to determine what's best for your body.

6 Nutritional Components that Fight Cancer

In the journey of fighting cancer naturally, understanding the nutritional components that have been shown to have cancer-fighting properties is crucial. This chapter will explore the roles of antioxidants, phytochemicals, and essential vitamins, along with specific foods that can enhance your diet and support your health.

Overview of Antioxidants

Antioxidants are compounds that help neutralize free radicals—unstable molecules that can damage cells and contribute to the development of cancer. By reducing oxidative stress in the body, antioxidants play a critical role in cancer prevention.

Key Types of Antioxidants:

- **Vitamin C**: A water-soluble vitamin that helps repair tissues and reduces inflammation.

- **Vitamin E**: A fat-soluble antioxidant that protects cell membranes from oxidative damage.

- **Selenium**: A trace mineral that contributes to antioxidant enzymes and immune function.

Overview of Phytochemicals

Phytochemicals are natural compounds found in plants that contribute to their color, flavor, and disease resistance. Many phytochemicals have been shown to have anti-cancer properties, supporting cellular health and reducing inflammation.

Key Categories:

- o **Flavonoids**: Found in fruits, vegetables, tea, and red wine; they possess strong antioxidant properties.

- o **Carotenoids**: Pigments found in carrots, sweet potatoes, and spinach; they have been linked to reduced cancer risk.

- o **Glucosinolates**: Present in cruciferous vegetables like broccoli and Brussels sprouts, these compounds may help detoxify carcinogens.

Specific Foods with Cancer-Fighting Properties

Certain foods are more effective at fighting cancer than others because of antioxidants, phytochemicals, and low acidity.

1. **Berries**:

   - o **Examples**: Blueberries, strawberries, and raspberries.

- o **Benefits**: Rich in antioxidants, particularly anthocyanins, which have been shown to inhibit cancer cell growth.

2. **Cruciferous Vegetables**:

    - o **Examples**: Broccoli, kale, cauliflower, and Brussels sprouts.

    - o **Benefits**: Contain glucosinolates that can activate detoxifying enzymes in the body and protect against cancer.

3. **Turmeric**:

    - o **Active Compound**: Curcumin.

    - o **Benefits**: Known for its anti-inflammatory and antioxidant properties, curcumin has shown promise in inhibiting cancer cell growth and promoting apoptosis (programmed cell death).

4. **Garlic**:

    - o **Benefits**: Contains organosulfur compounds that may help reduce the risk of certain cancers by enhancing immune function and inhibiting tumor growth.

5. **Green Tea**:

    - o **Active Component**: Epigallocatechin gallate (EGCG).

- o **Benefits**: A powerful antioxidant that has been associated with reduced risk of various cancers, particularly prostate and breast cancer.

6. **Tomatoes**:

   - o **Active Component**: Lycopene.

   - o **Benefits**: This antioxidant is more readily absorbed when tomatoes are cooked, and it has been linked to lower risk of prostate cancer.

7. **Nuts and Seeds**:

   - o **Examples**: Walnuts, flaxseeds, and chia seeds.

   - o **Benefits**: High in omega-3 fatty acids and antioxidants, these foods can help reduce inflammation and support overall health.

Next, let's explore, in depth, how integrating specific nutritional changes into your diet can potentially help reduce your body's acidity and inhibit further cancer growth.

6.1 The Role of Alkaline Water in Preventing Cancer

Alkaline water's benefits remain debated, but my personal experience showed it worked for me. When switching from acidic waters like Dasani or Aquafina to alkaline brands like Fiji or Essentia, the discomfort I had during urination disappeared, leading me to believe that alkaline water helped balance my body's pH and reduce acidity, a factor potentially linked to cancer development. In my humble opinion, it's worth the expense.

The Science Behind Alkalinity

While the body's kidneys and lungs naturally balance pH, some research suggests that creating an alkaline environment may inhibit cancer cell growth. Since our bodies are comprised of 60% water, alkaline water could be part of a preventative health strategy, but scientific consensus is still forming.

Many cultures have embraced alkaline water as part of their approach to cancer treatment. Asian countries, for instance—Japan, Hong Kong, and Singapore regularly make the list of the top ten places with the longest life spans globally. In contrast, no American city even breaks into the top 20. These countries often incorporate alkaline water into their healthcare practices, including cancer treatments. Perhaps they know something we haven't yet fully embraced in the West.

6.2 The Role of Vitamin C in Preventing Cancer

High-dose Vitamin C therapy has been hailed as a breakthrough treatment in the fight against cancer, particularly in intravenous form. According to Dr. Linus Pauling, a pioneer in this field, high doses of Vitamin C, when administered under the supervision of a healthcare professional, can induce cancer apoptosis—the process by which cancer cells self-destruct.

Although daily sources of Vitamin C are not as potent as high-dose Vitamin C therapy, they can still have a significant impact on the body.

List of Dietary Sources:

- **Lemons, Pineapples**: High in Vitamin C and antibacterial properties.

- **Mangoes, Oranges, Bell Peppers**: Rich in Vitamin C, supporting immune function and cancer prevention.

Juicing for Vitamin C

Daily juicing of fruits like mangoes, lemons, and blueberries, alongside regular consumption of avocados and bell peppers, helped me meet my daily Vitamin C intake while fighting cancer.

Dietary Vitamin C can also play a role in eliminating cancer cells. Citrus fruits like lemons and pineapples are known for their antibacterial properties, which can reduce cancer growth. While other fruits and vegetables, such as mangoes, oranges, and bell peppers, are also rich in Vitamin C, fewer studies have thoroughly examined their anti-cancer effects. Nevertheless, any fruit or vegetable containing high amounts of Vitamin C holds the potential to aid in reducing cancer cell proliferation.

Some patients undergoing high-dose Vitamin C therapy have gone into remission, while others have seen significant reductions in their tumor sizes, requiring less chemotherapy or surgical intervention. This cutting-edge treatment approach is one of the reasons I decided to embrace a vegetarian—or more precisely, a quasi-vegan—diet. I avoid dairy, eggs (except when they're baked into something), and cheese. To replace cheese, I sometimes use nutritional yeast, which provides a cheesy flavor without the dairy.

One of the primary ways I ensured I met my daily Vitamin C intake was through juicing. I enjoy blending fruits like mangoes, lemons, blueberries, pitaya, pineapples, and kiwi—all of which are high in Vitamin C and packed with cancer-fighting properties. I also made it a habit to eat an avocado and a bell pepper every day. These foods are rich in Vitamin C and contribute to the body's ability to combat cancer.

Whether you prefer juicing, making smoothies, eating fruits whole, or preparing vibrant breakfast bowls, incorporating Vitamin C-rich foods into your daily diet can help in the battle against cancer and other diseases. Besides targeting cancer cells, these foods also boost your immune system, helping to fight off colds and infections.

A Word of Caution

If you have diabetes or are monitoring your sugar intake, be cautious. Cancer and many other diseases feed on sugar. While refined sugar is the most problematic, even natural sugars from fruits can affect your body's delicate balance when you're fighting a disease. Experts often recommend a strict diet of leafy greens and other Vitamin C-rich vegetables to maximize health benefits without overloading on sugar.

Incorporating a variety of antioxidant-rich foods, phytochemicals, essential vitamins, and alkaline vitamins into your diet can significantly contribute to your cancer-fighting efforts. By focusing on whole, plant-based foods rich in these components, you can help support your body in its natural defenses against cancer.

In the next chapter, we will explore practical ways to implement these nutritional components into your daily meals and lifestyle, empowering you to take control of your health.

7 Creating Your Alkaline Diet Plan

Transitioning to an alkaline diet can seem daunting, but with a step-by-step guide, it can become an empowering part of your cancer-fighting journey. This chapter will provide practical strategies, sample meal plans, and shopping lists to help you create an effective alkaline diet plan.

Step-by-Step Guide to Transitioning to an Alkaline Diet

1. **Educate Yourself**:

    o Understand the principles of an alkaline diet. Familiarize yourself with alkaline-forming foods (fruits, vegetables, nuts, and seeds) and acid-forming foods (processed foods, sugars, and animal products).

2. **Evaluate Your Current Diet**:

    o Track your meals in a food diary for one week to assess your current eating habits. Record how frequently you consume acidic versus alkaline foods, and document how you feel after eating different foods.

3. **Set Realistic Goals**:

    o Start with small, achievable changes. Aim to incorporate one or two alkaline meals each week and gradually increase this over time.

- o If possible, try a one-week juice cleanse, ensuring that the juices are rich in iron to prevent light-headedness. As you reintroduce alkaline foods, document how they make you feel and whether they trigger any inflammation.

4. **Plan Your Meals**:

- o Use the sample meal plans provided in this chapter to create a balanced diet. Focus on variety to ensure you receive a wide range of nutrients.

- o Be mindful of your own allergies and intolerances and modify your diet accordingly. I have an intolerance to soy, and my reaction to edamame is immediate and severe. Soy lecithin, often found in chocolate bars, causes a milder reaction for me, but it's still uncomfortable. If I eat a small amount, my tongue burns, and I experience mild itching. However, if I indulge too much, I could have a major allergic reaction requiring medical attention.

  If you have allergies or intolerances— whether to gluten, soy, or any other food—steer clear of those allergens. Consuming foods that irritate your body weakens your immune system and can damage the lining of your intestines, preventing the proper absorption of essential nutrients. This makes it harder for your body to fight off diseases like cancer.

- o For those seeking sugar substitutes, Stevia leaf is a great option. It's natural, alkaline, and has a pH level of 10 or higher. However, be cautious with store-bought Stevia products, as many contain additives that may counteract your dietary goals. Honey, often praised for its antibacterial properties, can be helpful as well—though only pharmaceutical-grade Manuka honey has been proven effective in fighting cancer.

- o If you're diabetic and concerned about your sugar intake, there are fruits that can satisfy your nutritional needs without spiking your blood sugar. Lemons, tomatoes, avocados, dragon fruit (pitaya), and strawberries have some of the lowest sugar content among fruits. While it's important for diabetics to monitor all forms of sugar—whether natural or refined—these options provide a healthier alternative.

- o Always be mindful of what you put into your body. The foods you consume affect your immune system, your mood, and your overall well-being. Imagine how much less we'd rely on synthetic medications if we all ate fewer cookies, crackers, chips, breads, candy, and sugary drinks—and instead focused on fresh fruits and vegetables. Healthier dietary choices could make a world of difference.

5. **Create a Shopping List**:

- o Prepare a list of alkaline foods to stock your kitchen. Include fresh produce, whole grains, nuts, and seeds. Avoid processed foods and sugars.

6. **Cook and Prepare**:

- o Explore new recipes that focus on alkaline-rich foods. To save time during the week, try meal prepping. There are plenty of meal prep ideas available online—simply grab some bento boxes and mason jars to help organize your meals.

7. **Stay Hydrated**:

   o Drink plenty of alkaline-forming liquids, such as water with lemon or herbal teas, to support your body's detoxification processes.

8. **Monitor Your Progress**:

   o Keep track of how you feel as you transition. Note any changes in energy levels, mood, and overall health.

Sample Meal Plans

Sample Meal Plan for One Day

- **Breakfast**: Green smoothie with alkaline water, kale, green apples, avocado, cucumber, celery, kiwi, lemon juice, and chia seeds.

- **Snack**: A handful of pumpkin seeds and an apple.

- **Lunch**: Arugula salad with mixed greens, cherry tomatoes, cucumbers, and lemon-ginger dressing.

- **Snack**: Carrot and celery sticks with lemon or beet hummus.

- **Dinner**: Cauliflower steak with chimichurri over a bed of sauteed spinach and wild rice.

- **Dessert**: Chia seed pudding with berries and a drizzle of maple syrup.

Shopping List

- **Fruits**: Bananas, apples, berries, lemons, avocados.

- **Vegetables**: Spinach, kale, cauliflower, broccolini, bell peppers, carrots, cucumbers.

- **Whole Grains**: Wild rice (Quinoa may also work, but I am allergic. So, I typically avoid it)

- **Nuts and Seeds**: Pumpkin seeds, chia seeds, and flaxseeds. Almonds and walnuts are also somewhat alkaline, but I am allergic.

- **Herbs and Spices**: Ginger, garlic, turmeric, basil.

- **Oils**: Extra virgin olive oil and avocado oil. Coconut oil will work also, but I am allergic.

- **Beverages**: Alkaline water and green teas.

Part of your daily meal plan may also include juices. Juicing has gained attention for its potential to combat cancer, but the practice is not without controversy. Here are some key points of debate:

1. **Alkalinity**: Fresh juices, unless combined with alkaline-rich ingredients like lemons, limes, or bell peppers, can sometimes be more acidic than expected, which may not benefit the body's pH balance.

2. **Pasteurization**: Since fresh juices are not pasteurized, they can introduce harmful bacteria into the body, posing a risk for those with weakened immune systems.

3. **Loss of Nutrients**: The pulp of fruits and vegetables contains essential nutrients, especially fiber, which is lost during juicing. Fiber is a crucial component of a healthy diet.

Benefits of Juicing

1. **Faster Nutrient Absorption**: Juicing allows your body to absorb nutrients more efficiently since it bypasses the energy-intensive process of digesting whole fruits and vegetables.

2. **Alkalinity Support**: With the right combination of fruits and vegetables, juicing can help increase the body's alkalinity, promoting overall health.

3. **Detoxification**: Juicing aids in removing toxins and reducing inflammation. I personally enjoy adding cilantro and parsley to my juices for their detoxifying effects—cilantro is particularly good for eliminating harmful metals from the body.

My Favorite Cancer-Fighting Juices

1. **Green Detox** (Alkaline, Metal Detox, and Iron): Celery, chia seeds, kiwi, cilantro, garlic, cucumber, lemon, and lime.

2. **Green Immunity** (Iron, Immunity, Alkaline, and
   Metal Detox): Lemon, lime, collards, garlic, chia
   seeds, pineapple, cucumber, cilantro, parsley, red
   bell pepper, and mango.

3. **Vitamin C Boost** (Alkaline and Vitamin C):
   Lemon, lime, mango, and pineapple.

4. **Beets Cancer** (Alkalinity, Iron, and Cancer-
   Fighting Antioxidants): Beet roots and leaves,
   garlic, lemon, lime, celery, cucumber, chia seeds,
   and cilantro.

Choosing the Best Home Juicer

When selecting a juicer, you have two main options:
masticating and **centrifugal**.

- **Centrifugal Juicers**: These are more affordable
  and thus popular, but they operate at high speeds,
  which can result in the loss of important enzymes
  and nutrients due to the heat generated during the
  process.

- **Masticating Juicers**: Though more expensive,
  these juicers are a better investment for health-
  conscious individuals. They mimic the body's
  natural digestion process by grinding fruits and
  vegetables slowly, maximizing the retention of
  enzymes and nutrients. As a result, they are
  recommended over centrifugal juicers for those

seeking to extract the most health benefits from their produce.

8 Detoxification and Its Role in Healing

Detoxification is a vital aspect of supporting the body during cancer treatment and recovery. This chapter explores the importance of detoxifying the body and safe methods to complement an alkaline diet.

Importance of Detoxifying the Body During Cancer Treatment

1. **Eliminating Toxins:**

    o Cancer treatments, environmental pollutants, and dietary choices can lead to toxin accumulation in the body. Detoxification helps eliminate these harmful substances, promoting overall health.

2. **Enhancing Immune Function:**

    o A well-functioning detox system supports the immune response, which is crucial for fighting cancer and preventing recurrence.

3. **Improving Nutrient Absorption:**

    o Detoxification can enhance the body's ability to absorb nutrients from food, ensuring you receive the vitamins and minerals needed for healing.

4. **Reducing Inflammation:**

o   Many detox methods focus on reducing inflammation, which can help alleviate symptoms and improve the quality of life during cancer treatment.

Safe Detox Methods to Complement an Alkaline Diet

1. **Hydration**:

   Drinking ample water supports kidney function and helps flush out toxins. Aim for at least 8-10 glasses of alkaline water daily. Proper hydration is crucial for detoxification. Herbal teas and infused water with lemon or cucumber can also support hydration.

2. **Juicing**:

   Fresh vegetable and fruit juices can provide concentrated nutrients and antioxidants while aiding in detoxification. Incorporate fresh vegetable juices, particularly those high in greens and alkaline properties. Consider juices made with leafy greens, beets, and citrus fruits. A juice cleanse can help flush out toxins while providing essential nutrients.

3. **Herbal Teas**:

   Herbal teas such as dandelion, ginger, and green tea can support liver function and help with detoxification.

4. **Regular Exercise**:

Engaging in physical activity helps stimulate lymphatic flow and improve circulation, aiding in toxin elimination. Aim for a mix of aerobic exercises, strength training, and flexibility workouts, such as yoga.

5. **Deep Breathing and Relaxation Techniques**:

    Practices such as yoga, meditation, and deep breathing can reduce stress and promote detoxification by enhancing oxygen flow and reducing cortisol levels.

6. **Intermittent Fasting**

    Consider intermittent fasting to give your body a break from digestion, allowing it to focus on detoxification and cellular regeneration.

7. **Sauna and Sweat Therapy**:

    Using saunas can help open pores and promote sweating, a natural way to expel toxins from the body. During my battle with cancer, I used saunas daily for detox.

Integrating detoxification methods with an alkaline diet can significantly enhance your body's healing processes. By creating a comprehensive plan that includes nutritious foods and safe detox strategies, you empower yourself to take control of your health in the fight against cancer.

9 The Power of Hydration

Hydration plays a critical role in overall health and wellness, especially for those fighting cancer. This chapter explores the importance of water, particularly alkaline water, in cancer prevention and offers practical tips for staying hydrated and incorporating healthy beverages into your daily routine.

Role of Water and Alkaline Water in Cancer Prevention

1. **Maintaining Cellular Function**:

    o   Water is essential for cellular homeostasis, helping maintain balance in bodily functions. Adequate hydration supports nutrient absorption and waste elimination.

2. **Detoxification**:

    o   Water helps flush out toxins and metabolic waste, reducing the burden on the kidneys and liver. This detoxification process is vital for cancer patients as it aids in recovery and promotes a healthier environment for the body's cells.

3. **pH Balance**:

    o   Alkaline water, with a higher pH level than regular water, is believed to help neutralize acidity in the body. Some

studies suggest that an alkaline
environment may hinder cancer cell
growth, making alkaline water a
beneficial addition to your diet.

4. **Hydration and Energy Levels**:

   o Proper hydration is linked to improved
   energy levels and cognitive function.
   Staying hydrated can help combat fatigue,
   a common issue for those undergoing
   cancer treatment.

Tips for Staying Hydrated

1. **Set Daily Goals**:

   o Aim for at least 8-10 glasses of water per
   day. Adjust this based on your activity
   level, climate, and overall health.

2. **Infuse Your Water**:

   o Enhance the flavor and health benefits of
   your water by adding slices of fruits (like
   lemon, lime, or berries) or herbs (like
   mint or basil). This makes hydration more
   enjoyable.

3. **Incorporate Alkaline Beverages**:

   o Consider incorporating alkaline water or
   alkaline herbal teas into your routine.

Look for brands that offer natural alkaline water or invest in a water ionizer.

4. **Monitor Your Urine Color**:

   o A simple way to assess hydration levels is to monitor the color of your urine. Pale yellow indicates proper hydration, while darker shades suggest you may need to drink more water.

5. **Monitor Your Urine's pH**

   o Consider using pH strips to test your urine and monitor whether your pH levels are rising or falling. This will help you determine if your water intake and alkaline diet are effectively working for you.

6. **Healthy Beverage Choices**:

   o Explore other hydrating options such as herbal teas and homemade smoothies, ensuring they align with your alkaline diet goals.

Hydration is a powerful ally in your cancer-fighting journey. By prioritizing water and alkaline beverages, you can enhance your body's ability to heal and maintain optimal health.

10 The Alkaline Diet as a Complementary Approach

Given the potential risks associated with acidity from traditional treatments, the alkaline diet emerges as a promising complementary approach. Here's how it may help:

Restoring pH Balance

1. **Nutrient-Dense Foods**: The alkaline diet emphasizes consumption of fruits, vegetables, nuts, and seeds, which can help counteract acidity. These foods are rich in minerals like potassium and magnesium, which play a critical role in maintaining pH balance.

2. **Hydration and Detoxification**: An alkaline diet encourages adequate hydration through the consumption of alkaline water and hydrating foods. Proper hydration supports kidney function, aiding in the elimination of acidic waste products and promoting a more balanced pH.

Supporting Treatment Tolerance

1. **Mitigating Side Effects**: Patients adopting an alkaline diet often report fewer side effects from chemotherapy and radiation. The anti-inflammatory properties of alkaline foods may help reduce symptoms like nausea and fatigue, enhancing overall treatment tolerance.

2. **Promoting Recovery**: Nutritional support during
    and after cancer treatments is crucial for
    recovery. Alkaline foods rich in antioxidants can
    help repair cellular damage caused by treatments
    and promote cellular regeneration. This is
    particularly important for maintaining muscle
    mass and overall strength during treatment.

Enhancing Immune Function

By shifting to a more alkaline diet, patients may bolster
their immune function. The combination of increased
nutrient intake and reduced acidity can enhance the
activity of immune cells, which is especially beneficial
when the body is under the stress of cancer treatments.

The interplay between traditional cancer treatments and
body pH underscores the importance of dietary choices
in the overall management of cancer. While
chemotherapy and radiation can induce acidosis and its
associated risks, the alkaline diet offers a complementary
strategy to restore balance, mitigate side effects, and
support recovery. By integrating nutritional approaches
with conventional therapies, patients may enhance their
quality of life and improve treatment outcomes, fostering
a holistic approach to cancer care.

11 Lifestyle Changes for Optimal Health

Fighting cancer requires not only medical treatment but also significant lifestyle adjustments that promote holistic healing. Environmental factors, such as exposure to dust, chemicals, and everyday items like deodorants, toothpaste, and microwaves, may increase cancer risks. To mitigate these risks, reducing exposure to these toxins and using tools like air purifiers can create a cleaner environment, while simple remedies like apple cider vinegar may aid detoxification. Additionally, physical activity is essential. Engaging in aerobic exercises, strength training, and yoga helps improve circulation, support the immune system, and eliminate toxins through the lymphatic system.

Managing chronic stress, prioritizing quality sleep, and adopting mindful eating habits are equally important for those fighting cancer. Stress increases inflammation and acidity, both of which are linked to cancer progression. Techniques like meditation and deep breathing can help alleviate stress, while aiming for 7-9 hours of restorative sleep enhances the body's ability to detoxify and repair. Mindful eating, focused on whole, unprocessed foods and rich in alkaline-forming ingredients, supports the body at the cellular level and helps maintain pH balance. These strategies will also be discussed in detail throughout the chapter, highlighting their role in promoting overall well-being and cancer prevention.

Exercise plays a crucial role in helping cancer patients combat their illness and can reverse or control many other health conditions. It's widely acknowledged that regular physical activity aids in reducing cancer risk, and for those already diagnosed, it can significantly improve outcomes.

When I was diagnosed with cancer, I made exercise a daily priority. On most days, I walked between four to nine miles or aimed for 10,000 to 20,000 steps, driven by the belief that physical activity would help flush cancer from my body. These walks revitalized me. I felt more energetic, slept better at night, and experienced little to no sickness.

Studies show that exercise alone can reduce cancer risk dramatically. In fact, the World Health Organization (WHO) states that regular physical activity, along with maintaining a healthy body weight and diet, "can considerably reduce cancer risk." Healthy eating habits that prevent diet-related cancers also lower the risk of other noncommunicable diseases.

Exercise offers additional benefits to cancer patients, especially those undergoing chemotherapy. It helps alleviate fatigue and improves emotional well-being, aiding in the management of depression, anxiety, low self-esteem, and other factors that can affect a patient's quality of life.

Exercise offers additional benefits to cancer patients, especially those undergoing chemotherapy. It helps alleviate fatigue and improves emotional well-being, aiding in the management of depression, anxiety, low self-esteem, and other factors that can affect a patient's quality of life.

1. **Physical Activity Benefits**:

    o Regular exercise can improve physical strength, enhance immune function, and reduce fatigue. It is essential for maintaining a healthy weight and reducing the risk of cancer recurrence.

    o Exercise works in several ways to fight cancer. It lowers blood estrogen levels, which reduces a woman's risk of developing breast cancer. It also lowers insulin levels, creating an environment in which cancer cells are less likely to thrive. Beyond that, exercise triggers the production of natural killer (NK) cells. These NK cells, released when adrenaline is produced, target and destroy cancer cells.

    o I also enjoyed circuit training, which combined strength and endurance exercises into an intense, efficient workout. Here's an example of my circuit regimen:

1. TRX squats (five minutes)

2. Medicine ball exercises (five minutes)

3. Kettlebell squats and swings (five minutes)

4. Barbell squats (five minutes)

5. Rope arm exercises (five minutes)

6. Rest (five minutes) before repeating the circuit

2. **Recommended Activities**:

   o Aim for at least 150 minutes of moderate aerobic activity each week, such as brisk walking, swimming, or cycling. Incorporate strength training exercises at least twice a week.

   o Yoga became one of my favorite exercises. It's low impact but gets the blood flowing and adrenaline pumping. For cancer patients who feel anxious after a diagnosis, yoga's meditative aspect can help relieve stress. Personally, I found yoga to be both spiritually uplifting and physically effective.

3. **Listen to Your Body**:

- o Pay attention to how you feel during and after exercise. Modify your routine based on your energy levels and physical limitations.

- o After a particularly intense workout, I would punch a bag to release any pent-up anger, then hold a plank for three minutes. Once my session was done, I'd roll on a foam roller to stretch and relax my muscles. While most trainers recommend foam rolling before a workout, I preferred using it afterward. Rolling helped relieve soreness and alleviate pain caused by lactic acid buildup.

The type of exercise you choose is less important than the act of moving your body and keeping your adrenaline levels up. Remember, adrenaline triggers the production of natural killer cells, which are essential in the fight against cancer. Whether you prefer yoga, circuit training, walking, or something else entirely, staying active can help reduce feelings of depression and anxiety and boost your body's ability to fight back.

Many people pride themselves on functioning with minimal sleep. There's even a group known as the "sleepless elite" who boast about thriving on less than five hours a night. While this may sound impressive, have you ever considered the toll it might take on your body?

Research shows a strong link between inadequate sleep and cancer, as well as a range of other diseases, including heart disease, obesity, stroke, and diabetes. Excessive exposure to light at night is a significant factor contributing to sleep disturbances. Stress and anxiety also play major roles in sleepless nights. With over 70 percent of Americans getting less than the recommended eight hours of sleep each night, it's no surprise that heart disease and cancer rank among the leading causes of death in the U.S.

Bodybuilders often recognize that rest and sleep are just as crucial for muscle development as workouts. During sleep, the body repairs itself and produces melatonin, a hormone that plays a vital role in fighting cancer. Adequate sleep is essential if your primary goal is to achieve cancer remission.

Melatonin is secreted only when you sleep in a dark environment. Sleeping in a well-lit room inhibits its production. In 1987, researcher Richard G. Stevens published findings in the *American Journal of Epidemiology* that demonstrated how circadian disruption can hinder melatonin production, which is a potent antioxidant that combats cancer. Women who produce less melatonin show higher rates of breast cancer. Interestingly, studies found that blind women who lived in darkness and slept more frequently had significantly lower incidences of breast cancer compared to their sighted counterparts. Lower melatonin levels correlate with increased estrogen production, and high estrogen levels are linked to the growth of breast cancer. Melatonin, often referred to as the "darkness hormone," is essential for fighting free radicals that promote cancer growth.

Cortisol, another crucial hormone, also plays a role in cancer prevention. It bolsters the immune system and acts as an antioxidant, helping to prevent the formation of free radicals. Research indicates that cortisol levels increase in proportion to the amount of sleep one gets each night. Individuals with lower cortisol levels tend to have shorter lifespans than those with higher levels.

Dr. David Spiegel at Stanford University corroborated Stevens' findings in a study involving women and shift work. He noted that women engaged in shift work faced higher incidences of breast cancer, attributing this to the "light at night" phenomenon that disrupts normal sleep patterns. The World Health Organization has even suggested that shift work may contribute to increased rates of cancer and obesity.

If you struggle with nighttime light, consider investing in blackout curtains or using a dim red light to promote better sleep. For those dealing with anxiety or stress, regular exercise, meditation, and healthy eating can help alleviate these issues. If sleep problems persist, consulting a physician may be necessary to address specific concerns.

Physical activity can counteract the negative effects of sedentary lifestyles, making it easier to fall asleep. Many people who stand or move throughout the day find it easier to drift off at night because their bodies are genuinely fatigued.

While Stevens doesn't recommend artificial melatonin supplements, he advocates for natural sleep as the optimal treatment. Remember, a completely dark room is crucial for producing sufficient melatonin. Use only dim red light if necessary and avoid screens—televisions and phones—before bed. Ensuring a dark environment is vital for cancer prevention and reduction.

Throughout my cancer journey, I managed to sleep eight hours or more most of the time. Some years, I consistently achieved this, while other nights I averaged five to seven hours, often waking several times. I believe that adequate sleep played a significant role in helping my immune system fight off cancer cells, ultimately contributing to my cancer-free diagnosis.

Here are some other sleep tips that may help:

1. **Restorative Sleep**:

    o   Quality sleep is essential for healing and
        recovery. It allows your body to repair
        and regenerate, supporting overall health.

2. **Sleep Hygiene Tips**:

    o   Establish a regular sleep schedule by
        going to bed and waking up at the same
        time each day. Create a calming bedtime
        routine and ensure your sleeping
        environment is comfortable and dark.

3. **Limit Stimulants**:

    o   Avoid caffeine, nicotine, and heavy meals
        close to bedtime. Instead, opt for calming
        herbal teas to promote relaxation.

Managing stress is an essential aspect of supporting the body during cancer treatment. Chronic stress negatively impacts the immune system, weakens the body's defense mechanisms, and contributes to inflammation—factors that can impede recovery and even exacerbate disease progression. By effectively managing stress, cancer patients can promote healing, improve treatment outcomes, and enhance overall well-being.

Holistic stress-management practices, such as yoga, meditation, and deep breathing exercises, have been shown to lower cortisol levels and reduce anxiety. These techniques also help cultivate emotional resilience, which is important during the physically and mentally demanding process of cancer treatment. Engaging in such practices regularly can help maintain emotional stability, which supports a more balanced, healing environment within the body.

In addition to structured practices, mindfulness techniques—such as journaling, guided imagery, and simply being present in the moment—can further alleviate stress. These practices encourage self-awareness and reduce the mind's tendency to dwell on fear or uncertainty. By managing stress holistically, cancer patients can improve their quality of life and create a supportive atmosphere for recovery.

Here's a synopsis and a reminder of the importance of stress management:

1. **Impact of Stress on Health**:

   o   Chronic stress can negatively affect your immune system and overall well-being. Managing stress is crucial for maintaining health during cancer treatment.

2. **Holistic Practices**:

   o   Incorporate practices like yoga, meditation, and deep breathing exercises into your daily routine. These can help reduce stress levels and promote emotional well-being.

3. **Mindfulness Techniques**:

   o   Practice mindfulness by being present in the moment. Techniques such as journaling or guided imagery can also help in managing stress and anxiety.

Implementing lifestyle changes can significantly impact your health and well-being during your cancer journey. By prioritizing exercise, quality sleep, and stress management techniques, you empower yourself to enhance your overall quality of life.

11.4 Importance of Understanding Allergies, Immunity, and Cancer: A Complex Relationship

Allergic reactions can weaken the immune system. The histamine response may release hormones, free radicals, or promote chronic inflammation, potentially encouraging the development of cancer. While one study has suggested this correlation, conclusive evidence is lacking.

Interestingly, I discovered that some research indicates individuals with cancer may have lower levels of IgE and overall allergies—contrary to what I had previously understood. This complicates the discussion around the relationship between allergies and cancer, making it challenging to draw definitive conclusions.

Personally, I've experienced both cancer and numerous allergies. I'm allergic to smoke, dust, cats, dogs, pests, soy, wheat, nuts, gluten, quinoa, and shrimp. I was diagnosed with most of these allergies in 1999, but after my cancer diagnosis, soy, dairy, eggs, quinoa, and shrimp were added to the list. My situation doesn't seem to align with the findings of that study, suggesting that many factors beyond cancer may contribute to the development of adult-onset allergies.

Some research posits that individuals with allergies may fight cancer more effectively. When the immune system detects allergens like dust or pollen, it triggers an immune response, preparing the body to combat potential threats. In contrast, individuals without allergies might not mount a strong immune response because cancer cells often disguise themselves as normal cells. Allergic reactions can unmask these cancer cells and activate natural killer cells, making allergies potentially beneficial in this context.

A 2007 article in the *Journal of Epidemiology* suggested that allergies might lower the risk of developing brain cancer, offering some hope for allergy sufferers like me. Additionally, an NIH article indicated that those with allergies may be less likely to be diagnosed with cancer, as the immune response triggered by allergies helps eliminate cancer-causing free radicals, aligning with previous findings.

On the flip side, some studies have linked cancer to allergies. A 1992 study found that men with drug allergies had a 33 percent higher risk of developing cancer, while women with drug allergies showed a 21 percent decrease in risk. However, research also suggested that individuals with a history of allergies might be at greater risk for prostate and breast cancer.

Further research has shown that people with eczema and asthma are more likely to develop blood and lung cancers. I had eczema and rheumatoid arthritis as a child, which points to a potentially weak immune system and a higher propensity for these types of cancer. A 2003 study also indicated a connection between allergies to trees, grass, and plants and blood cancers.

A 2015 study published in the *Journal of Leukocyte Biology* noted that pulmonary inflammation could elevate cancer risk, while another study indicated that chronic inflammation is a known risk factor for cancer. Research from 2014 established a link between histamines and cancer, suggesting that histamines might protect tumors, complicating the ability of natural killer cells to identify and eliminate cancer cells.

Experts have suggested that allergy shots and medications might target and destroy cancer cells, which contradicts what I had previously read—that allergy medications could increase cancer risk. It's possible that this only applies to certain over-the-counter medications. More investigation is needed, and I plan to share my findings in the future.

While the relationship between allergies and cancer remains complex, being aware of how allergies might influence cancer risk is enlightening. I always assumed that allergies could increase cancer risk, so it's reassuring to learn they might also aid in prevention.

11.5 Meat, Cancer, and the Truth: Why Eliminating Processed Foods Matters

Americans have a deep love for bacon and sausage. During President Obama's administration, a Hawaiian food revival emerged, but it is to the detriment of cancer patients. A diet heavy in pork and Spam isn't recommended for those battling cancer.

My maternal grandmother was no stranger to the Spam and pork diet; she relished it and prepared it frequently during my childhood. Breakfast at her house was a hearty affair—bacon, eggs, sausage, pancakes, and grits graced the table every single morning, seven days a week. While I preferred grits and cold cereal, the rest of the family indulged, and they all struggled with their weight. I often attributed my own slenderness to being more active, but it likely stemmed from my food choices as well.

Though my grandma was never diagnosed with cancer, she did suffer from severe arthritis, which can be worsened by a diet high in processed meats. While I cherish those memories, I can't help but wonder if her dietary choices impacted her health negatively.

Research shows that any processed meat, including sausage, bacon, and deli meats, increases cancer risk. In fact, some studies suggest that consuming these products may be as harmful as smoking. According to the World Health Organization (WHO) in 2015, hot dogs, sausages, processed deli meats, ham, and bacon are linked to cancer development. Additionally, both beef and pork are included in these findings. Notably, some studies suggest that eating eggs can significantly increase prostate cancer risk in men—by as much as 81 percent if they consume 2.5 eggs per week.

For those concerned about cancer, adopting a diet free from animal products may be the best course of action. This recommendation extends to yogurt, dairy, eggs, and all types of meat. If you must consume meat, wild fish is the healthiest option, and grass-fed beef is preferable to conventionally raised beef. Overall, processed meats pose a greater risk than traditional cuts. A plant-based, whole foods diet is highly recommended.

Foods to Avoid if You're Battling Cancer:

- Processed meats

- Microwave popcorn

- French fries

- Potato chips

- Hydrogenated oils containing trans fats

- Farmed salmon

- Soda

- Foods made with refined sugar

For me, refined sugar has been the biggest challenge. I struggled to give up my beloved Hershey's Kisses and chocolate bars. As a healthier alternative, I turned to 85 percent dark chocolate by Lindt, though cocoa still poses some acidity issues.

Eliminating processed meats, farmed salmon, potato chips, and French fries was relatively easy for me. I hadn't consumed soda since I was a child, save for the occasional ginger ale when I felt nauseated. Overall, cutting these items from my diet was a manageable, albeit necessary, transition.

11.6 The Importance of Apple Cider Vinegar: A Natural Ally in the Fight Against Cancer

Apple cider vinegar (ACV) is renowned for its numerous health benefits, particularly its antibacterial properties and its ability to promote an alkaline environment in the body. For individuals facing cancer, raw apple cider vinegar is often the only type of vinegar recommended.

Unlike other vinegars—such as white wine vinegar, red wine vinegar, balsamic vinegar, and white vinegar—which are acid-forming and may contribute to an environment conducive to cancer growth, raw apple cider vinegar is considered an optimal choice for those concerned about both cancer and maintaining a balanced pH level.

Incorporating raw apple cider vinegar into your diet may offer not only potential health benefits but also a simple way to support your overall well-being during challenging times. However, as with any dietary change, it's essential to consult with healthcare professionals to ensure it aligns with your treatment plan and personal health needs.

11.7 Air Quality Matters: How Purifiers Help Create a Safer Healing Environment

During my battle with cancer, I decided to use an air purifier to help cleanse my environment of potential carcinogens. I had read that indoor air quality can be just as detrimental to health as outdoor air quality. So, I kept the purifier running while I worked to filter out airborne allergens and pollutants.

While I can't say for certain how much it contributed to my recovery, I figured it was worth a shot. I used a Holmes air purifier, which performed well in a small room. I found it to be a reliable brand.

Experts often recommend using an air purifier equipped with both a HEPA filter and a UV light. These models are designed to eliminate airborne viruses, mold, and fungi—threats that can significantly compromise a weakened immune system. For cancer patients, an air purifier can help reduce the risk of infections from airborne pathogens.

11.8 The Hidden Dangers of Dust: A Silent Threat to Your Health

As someone who is allergic to dust, I've developed a keen interest in the hidden dangers it poses. Research reveals that household dust often contains a variety of toxic chemicals linked to cancer, infertility, and developmental issues in children. Among the most concerning substances are phthalates, which can be found in everything from beauty products to vinyl flooring.

Dust is not just a nuisance; it can be a cocktail of harmful chemicals shed from electrical goods, cleaning products, and even the flooring itself. We often think our homes are safe havens, but indoor air pollution from dust can be just as dangerous as outdoor pollution.

Many parents allow their babies and young children to play on the floor without realizing the potential risks. Children frequently put their hands in their mouths, and even tiny amounts of toxic dust can harm their developing bodies.

A study published in the *Journal of Environmental Science and Technology* identified over 45 toxic chemicals in dust collected from homes, schools, and gyms. Alarmingly, 90 percent of the samples contained ten of the most common toxic substances, including flame retardants and phenols. For example, the flame retardant TDCIPP, found in baby products, carpet padding, and furniture foam, has been linked to cancer risk.

Phthalates, another group of harmful chemicals, are prevalent in personal care products and food packaging, raising concerns about hormone disruption and reproductive problems. Disturbingly, they're even found in beloved foods like Kraft Macaroni and Cheese, a staple in many households.

Further research has shown that the number of toxins in household dust often exceeds EPA standards, highlighting the urgent need for awareness and action to protect our families.

To mitigate these risks, you should actively reduce dust levels in your home. Here are some practical steps:

1. **Wash Hands Regularly**: Use plain soap and water to keep hands clean, especially before meals.

2. **Regular Cleaning**: Sweep and mop floors regularly to minimize dust accumulation. Also, clean and disinfect all surfaces including doorknobs, telephones, chargers, kitchen tables, baseboards, countertops and living room and bedroom furniture.

3. **Natural Cleaners**: Consider using natural cleaning substances like lemon and vinegar, enhanced with essential oils like citronella,

rosemary, or lavender, to disinfect without harsh chemicals.

While bleach can be effective for germ reduction, it must be used cautiously due to its potential harm if inhaled or ingested over time. Although there's no definitive evidence linking bleach to cancer, it's wise to explore safer alternatives.

Don't forget to vacuum frequently and dust surfaces to keep your home clean. If you have carpets, consider shampooing them at least once every two weeks or once a month. I cleaned my carpets once a week, and it improved my health.

Experts suggest that the risks posed by toxic dust contamination outweigh concerns of developing allergies from overly sterile environments. I share this belief—maintaining a clean home not only improves mood but also fosters clarity of thought.

By being proactive about dust management, we can help safeguard our families against these hidden threats.

11.9 The Silent Threats of Old Construction: Protecting Your Health in Aging Buildings

Just as we learned that dust contains toxins, we must also be cognizant of the risks in older construction homes. It's alarming to see cancer patients living in older homes, often unaware of the carcinogenic risks lurking within.

When I was battling cancer, I was acutely conscious of avoiding old construction, knowing that exposure to harmful substances could significantly impact my health. Some of the key risks associated with older buildings include:

1. **Asbestos**

2. **Silica**

3. **Wood Dust**

4. **Certain Paints and Solvents**

Homes built before the 1970s, particularly those from the late 1800s and early 1900s, are more likely to contain asbestos. This once-popular insulation material was valued for its fire resistance, but its glass-like fibers can cause serious lung diseases, including lung cancer and mesothelioma, often decades after initial exposure.

Research indicates that individuals exposed to asbestos may not show symptoms of lung cancer until 20 years later, by which time the prognosis can be dire. Some patients often have only a few months to live after diagnosis. Therefore, those who have been exposed should seek annual checkups to monitor their health.

Additionally, older homes may harbor dust laden with carcinogens and lead-based paints, posing further health risks. Cancer patients and their loved ones should advocate for newer construction to minimize these hazards and improve health outcomes. For anyone supporting someone with cancer, it's crucial not to push them into environments that could exacerbate their condition.

While asbestos has been banned in new construction in the U.S. since the 1970s, many older buildings still contain it. If you suspect exposure, it's vital to consult a doctor immediately to explore preventive measures.

In my view, any home built before the 1990s should be considered for rebuilding, and communities should focus on modern, safe construction practices. I recognize that some may view this stance as extreme, but I firmly believe that all buildings should adhere to clean EPA and LEED standards. Advocating for such measures, along with eliminating BPAs in food packaging, is essential for safeguarding our health and the health of future generations.

11.10 Natural Alternatives: Reducing Cancer Risks with Eco-Friendly Cleaners

Numerous studies suggest a troubling connection between cleaning chemicals and cancer. The *Journal of Environmental Health* has reported that certain cleaning products may be linked to cancer in the mammary glands. Some of the key carcinogens to be aware of include:

1. **Methylene Chloride**

2. **Nitrobenzene**

Just as working with specific solvents can elevate cancer risks, so too can everyday cleaning products. For those undergoing cancer treatment, many health professionals recommend natural cleaning solutions, such as vinegar and lemon, to avoid potential complications.

Several brands, like Eco-Clean and Bentley Organic, are recognized for producing cleaning products that contain little or no toxic substances. Vinegar-based cleaners—whether homemade or sourced from eco-friendly advocates—represent some of the safest, toxin-free options currently available. In addition to the known carcinogens, there are other chemicals of concern that require further research before being classified as carcinogenic. These include:

1. **Phthalates**

2. **Ammonia**

3. **Sodium Hydroxide**

4. **Triclosan**

5. **Chlorine**

6. **Perchloroethylene (PERC)**

7. **Quaternary Ammonium Compounds (QUATS)**

8. **N2-Butoxyethylene**

During my own cancer journey, I found it essential to minimize the burden of cleaning for others. I relied on a maid service half the time and managed my own cleaning once a week. If hiring a cleaning service is feasible, consider scheduling them every week or every two weeks. If you can afford it, I recommend hiring someone four times a week. In between professional cleanings, it's crucial to keep surfaces disinfected to prevent toxin accumulation.

Investing in a cleaning service that uses natural products is, in my humble opinion, a worthwhile expenditure for anyone diagnosed with cancer. Your health should always be a priority, and taking proactive steps to ensure a toxin-free environment can make a significant difference.

11.11 Misconceptions About Cannabis, Health and the Carcinogenic Nature of All Smoke

It's common knowledge that smoking causes cancer—it's even printed on cigarette packages. Yet, I've seen countless individuals continue to smoke during chemotherapy or other cancer treatments. Smoke from any source—whether it's a tobacco cigarette, incense, marijuana, or even smoke from wood-burning stoves and barbecues—is detrimental to your health and often carcinogenic. Even burning olive oil can release harmful substances.

All smoke contains carbon monoxide, carbon dioxide, and particulate matter (PM or soot). It can also contain a variety of chemicals, including aldehydes, acid gases, sulfur dioxide, nitrogen oxides, polycyclic aromatic hydrocarbons (PAHs), benzene, toluene, styrene, metals, and dioxins. The specific particles and chemicals present depend on what is burning, the oxygen available, and the burn temperature.

According to the American Lung Association, "Smoke is harmful to lung health. Whether from burning wood, tobacco, or marijuana, toxins and carcinogens are released during combustion. Smoke from marijuana combustion has been shown to contain many of the same toxins, irritants, and carcinogens as tobacco smoke."

So, it's misguided to think that marijuana cigarettes are a cure for cancer. Smoke is still inhaled into your lungs and is likely to contribute to cancer development.

I once knew someone who regularly inhaled marijuana smoke. Despite exercising constantly and following a vegetarian diet that included collards, tomatoes, and kale, he still developed prostate cancer. Inhaling any kind of smoke is detrimental to health.

To be fair, he also rarely got more than five hours of sleep per night and had a diet loaded with pizza, Oreos, and Cheez-Its, particularly pizza, which is high in acidity due to its wheat and cheese content. These choices were far from healthy. Oreos are full of refined sugar, and Cheez-Its are heavily processed. While kale and collards may have slowed cancer growth, they weren't enough to counteract the free radicals introduced by his diet of pizza, fries, and marijuana cigarettes.

Another acquaintance of mine barbequed at least four times a week. Later, he developed throat and mouth cancer. This exposure to smoke may have contributed to producing an environment where cancer could grow in the body.

While cannabis oil shows some promise in cancer treatment, the results are mixed, and its effectiveness remains inconclusive. One thing is clear: you don't need the THC-induced "high" to combat cancer. This raises questions about the validity of arguments supporting recreational marijuana use.

In my own cancer journey, I've never smoked marijuana or used any illegal or legal street drugs. I managed to overcome cancer without them, and I believe you can too.

To be candid, I developed cervical cancer after dating a smoker. Experts assert that secondhand smoke can be deadly, and women who smoke are at a higher risk for cervical cancer. Although I never smoked myself, being involved with a smoker and having intimate relations with a promiscuous partner likely contributed to my diagnosis.

I'm allergic to smoke and actively avoid living with smokers, frequenting smoky bars or casinos, or dating smokers. Exposure to smoke is harmful and may significantly increase the risk of developing cancer.

11.12 The Hidden Dangers of Hair Care: Chemicals and Cancer Risk

For years, experts have warned that professions like hairstyling and construction carry an increased risk of cancer. The fumes and chemicals found in products like formaldehyde-based treatments, keratin, hair dyes, and chemical straighteners can contribute to this heightened risk.

During my cancer battle, I made the difficult decision to limit my salon visits to just once a year for a trim, color, and blowout. As someone who typically enjoyed weekly appointments, this change was challenging. However, I was determined to prioritize my health and work within my modest budget, willing to try anything that might help.

Research published in the *International Journal of Epidemiology* supports the concern, revealing that hair stylists face a significantly higher cancer risk than the general population. Experts recommend that salons maintain optimal ventilation systems and adopt improved hygiene practices to help mitigate these risks.

While I can't say for certain that my reduced salon visits made a difference, I felt it was a necessary precaution during a critical time in my life.

Recent advancements in hair care have made it simpler to achieve a stylish look while minimizing exposure to harmful chemicals and smoke from styling tools. For instance, using mousse and flexirods can create curls without heat, while collagen treatments offer a safer alternative for straightening hair compared to traditional relaxers. Additionally, the trend of embracing baldness, popularized by celebrities like Jada Pinkett Smith, has made going bald a fashionable choice. With these innovations and a shift in societal norms, cancer patients can prioritize their beauty routines without the risk of cancer-related exposure.

11.13 BPA and Beyond: Understanding Canned Food Risks

In our fast-paced society, convenience and disaster preparedness often trumps health, and canned foods exemplify this trend. While they offer time-saving benefits, the risks associated with them, particularly the presence of BPAs (bisphenol-A), can outweigh the convenience. These chemicals, commonly found in the lining of canned foods, have been linked to an increased cancer risk.

The canning process itself can diminish some nutritional value, but BPAs are a significant reason to reconsider reaching for that can. Classified as endocrine disruptors by experts like Dr. Ana Soto from Tufts University School of Medicine, BPAs have shown a potential link to cancer growth in animal studies, although definitive proof of their impact on human cancer remains elusive due to ethical constraints in research.

A 2017 study by the Center for Environmental Health evaluated cans from major retailers and found that 40% contained cancer-associated BPAs. While alarming, this is an improvement from the 67% found two years prior. Further studies indicated that over 2,500 participants who regularly consumed canned foods had detectable BPA levels in their urine—an unsettling statistic given the known carcinogenic properties of BPAs.

For me, the implications of these findings were enough to eliminate canned foods from my diet, except in

emergencies like natural disasters, where canned goods
are invaluable for their durability and safety from
contamination.

Microwaves often face criticism for depleting nutrients in food and potentially increasing cancer risk. However, research from the Cancer Council NSW and the American Cancer Society offers a different perspective.

According to their findings, "Microwave ovens do not make foods radioactive. They heat food by producing radiation that is absorbed by water molecules, causing them to vibrate and generate heat. This process cooks the food without altering its chemical structure in a way that increases cancer risk. If used correctly, microwaves have no known harmful effects on humans."

During my initial years battling cancer, I frequently relied on the microwave. While studies suggest it's safe, I noticed something unsettling about how I felt after eating microwaved food, though I couldn't pinpoint the cause.

Eventually, I decided to shift away from microwave meals, opting instead for salads, cold beans, raw vegetables, or stovetop-cooked dishes. There's a lot of debate around this topic, but I observed that consuming microwaved canned food often left me with a low-grade headache. Perhaps it was the BPA in the cans, but whatever the reason, it was an uncomfortable sensation. Therefore, I lean towards the idea that avoiding microwave dinners while fighting cancer could be beneficial.

The American Cancer Society states, "Microwave ovens do not use x-rays or gamma rays, and they do not make food radioactive. While they can cook food effectively, they do not alter its chemical or molecular structure. Microwaves are designed to be contained within the oven, and if they are used properly, there's no evidence they pose health risks. In the U.S., strict federal standards limit radiation leakage to levels far below those that could cause harm. However, damaged or modified ovens might allow microwaves to leak, potentially leading to burns."

From my personal experience, it seemed that microwave dinners negatively impacted me. During a transitional phase in my life, I consumed them regularly and often felt faint, even blacking out at least once a day with no recollection of those moments. This alarming pattern persisted for a month until I ended up in the emergency room. While they didn't check my iron levels, I suspect they were low. The doctors attributed my episodes to syncope and mild dehydration.

After I stopped eating microwave dinners, the fainting spells ceased. My water intake didn't change significantly, so eliminating those meals seemed to play a crucial role in my recovery. While factors like frozen food, inadequate hydration, or low iron might have contributed to my symptoms, it's always wise to err on the side of caution when it comes to diet, especially during a cancer journey.

11.15 Daily Habits: Are Your Toothpaste Choices Putting You at Risk?

Recent studies have raised concerns about certain ingredients in toothpaste, particularly titanium dioxide. This compound, commonly found in many dental products, has been linked to precancerous growths. In a study conducted in France and Luxembourg, over 40% of lab rats given titanium dioxide in their drinking water developed cancerous tumors. This ingredient, often labeled as E171, is also present in a variety of consumer products, including chocolates, sweets, sunscreen, and gum.

Another ingredient of concern is Triclosan, a common antimicrobial agent found in many beauty and personal care products. A 2016 study highlighted its potential dangers, showing that Triclosan may be as harmful as titanium dioxide. Despite these findings, the FDA has not banned Triclosan from Colgate Total toothpaste, citing its proven effectiveness in reducing gum inflammation and plaque. However, its presence raises questions about possible contributions to cancer growth, prompting advocates to push for its removal.

A significant study published in the *Journal Proceedings of the National Academy of Sciences* by researchers from the University of California at San Diego and the University of California at Davis revealed that introducing Triclosan into lab rats with pre-existing tumors led to increased tumor size. This suggests that

Triclosan may act as a hormone disruptor and contribute to antibiotic resistance.

Toothpaste is a product we use daily, and I must admit that despite these concerns, I didn't change mine during my cancer battle. I have a fondness for Procter & Gamble's Crest and switching to more natural alternatives like charcoal or baking soda has been challenging for me. We all have our weaknesses, and toothpaste happens to be mine. Perhaps I should consider making my own.

While I successfully fought cancer without altering my toothpaste routine, I encourage others to consider their choices carefully. Eliminating environmental carcinogens from your life can only improve your health and prognosis.

11.16 Natural Alternatives: Rethinking Deodorant Choices in the Age of Cancer Awareness

As a kid, deodorant was a must-have, but even with antiperspirants, I often felt like nothing really worked. My struggles with excessive sweating and odor didn't improve until I removed allergens from my diet and environment. I discovered that when I consumed allergen-rich foods or was exposed to environmental triggers, I would sweat more and emit stronger odors. Foods like meat, processed items, and refined sugars exacerbated the problem.

Now, armed with this knowledge, I can comfortably go deodorant-free during the winter and for most of the summer. I suspect hormonal changes as I age may also play a role in this shift.

On warmer days, I prefer to keep things natural and toxin-free. Sometimes, I use lime as a deodorant or opt for products with fewer aluminum compounds and parabens, which are often the focus of concerns linking deodorants and antiperspirants to cancer. Many people recommend brands like Native for those seeking a more natural alternative.

According to the American Cancer Society, as of 2014, there's no conclusive evidence that aluminum or parabens in deodorants cause cancer. They consider it acceptable to use deodorants containing aluminum for now. However, ongoing research may yield new insights in the future.

12 Mindset and Mental Well-Being

The connection between mental health and physical health is profound, especially when fighting cancer. This chapter explores the importance of maintaining a positive mindset and provides techniques to nurture mental well-being during treatment.

The Connection Between Mental Health and Physical Health

1. **Psychosomatic Relationship**:

While the National Cancer Institute states that there is no conclusive evidence linking stress directly to cancer, I believe that poorly managed stress can weaken the immune system and trigger the release of hormones that may contribute to cancer development.

Stress can lead to sleepless nights, and inadequate sleep can reduce melatonin production. Although there may not be a direct correlation, stress certainly increases the likelihood of behaviors that can promote cancer growth. It's important to recognize the impact of stress on overall health and to find effective ways to manage it.

Mental health directly impacts physical health. Stress, anxiety, and depression can weaken the immune system, making it harder for the body to fight cancer.

2. **Emotional Resilience**:

Building emotional resilience helps individuals cope with the challenges of cancer treatment. A positive mindset can improve quality of life and even influence treatment outcomes.

3. **Mind-Body Connection**:

Practices such as meditation and visualization can enhance the mind-body connection, promoting healing and reducing stress.

Techniques for Maintaining a Positive Mindset

During my battle with cancer, I found solace in meditation. I often expressed gratitude for the simple things in life—a roof over my head, my car, which I cherished like a best friend. Losing my car was difficult, and I prayed for the day I could thank God for a stable home, health insurance, and even a vacation. I believe that practicing gratitude can help release some of the anger that often accompanies a cancer diagnosis.

My anger was compounded by the trauma of sexual assault, which I felt played a role in my illness. Through meditation and singing gospel music from my childhood, I kept my spirits up while working in a job unrelated to my education. Daily meditation and yoga became essential tools for maintaining my motivation and emotional health, and I truly think they made a difference.

Research supports the benefits of mindfulness. A study titled "Mindfulness-based cancer recovery and supportive-expressive therapy maintain telomere length relative to controls in distressed breast cancer survivors" found that participants showed increased cortisol levels, which help combat free radicals and cancer. However, it also revealed decreased telomere length in the control group, indicating a potential impact on cancer prognosis.

This study is among the first to provide conclusive evidence that meditation and Hatha yoga can positively influence cortisol levels and potentially cancer growth compared to a control group that did not engage in these practices.

As I've always said, meditation cannot hurt you. Even if it doesn't directly reduce cancer growth, it can enhance your mood and alleviate stress. I tried it, and it helped me immensely, so I wholeheartedly recommend it to others facing similar challenges.

1. **Gratitude Practice**:

    o Start a daily gratitude journal to reflect on positive experiences and things you're thankful for. This practice can shift focus from negativity to appreciation.

2. **Affirmations**:

    o Use positive affirmations to reinforce a hopeful outlook. Phrases like "I am strong" or "I am healing" can be powerful tools to combat negative thoughts.

3. **Mindfulness and Meditation**:

   o Engage in mindfulness practices to remain present and reduce anxiety. Consider guided meditation apps or local classes to help you get started.

4. **Visualization Techniques**:

   o Visualize your body healing and overcoming cancer. This can create a sense of empowerment and enhance your emotional resilience.

5. **Seek Professional Help**:

   o Don't hesitate to seek support from a mental health professional. Therapists or counselors can provide valuable tools and coping strategies during this challenging time.

Maintaining a positive mindset is essential in the fight against cancer. By incorporating techniques that foster mental well-being, you can empower yourself to face challenges with resilience and hope. The next chapter will focus on the vital role of support systems and community in navigating your cancer journey.

13 Support Systems and Community

Having a robust support network is crucial for those battling cancer. This chapter discusses the importance of community and how to find groups and resources that can provide valuable assistance and connection.

Importance of Having a Support Network

1. **Emotional Support**:

   o Friends, family, and community members provide emotional support, helping to alleviate feelings of isolation and fear. Their encouragement can boost your morale during treatment.

2. **Practical Help**:

   o Support networks can also offer practical assistance, such as meal preparation, transportation to appointments, or help with household tasks, allowing you to focus on healing.

3. **Shared Experiences**:

   o Connecting with others who have faced similar challenges can provide comfort and understanding. Sharing experiences can foster a sense of camaraderie and hope.

Finding Groups and Resources for Cancer Patients

1. **Local Support Groups**:

   o   Look for local cancer support groups
       through hospitals, cancer centers, or
       community organizations. These groups
       often host meetings where patients can
       share their experiences and coping
       strategies.

2. **Online Communities**:

   o   Online platforms and forums can connect
       you with others facing cancer. Websites
       like Cancer Support Community and
       forums on social media can provide a
       wealth of information and emotional
       support.

3. **Nonprofit Organizations**:

   o   Many nonprofits focus on cancer support,
       offering resources such as counseling,
       financial assistance, and educational
       materials. Research organizations like the
       American Cancer Society for resources
       specific to your needs.

4. **Peer Mentorship Programs**:

   o   Some organizations provide mentorship
       programs that pair newly diagnosed
       patients with survivors. These

relationships can be incredibly beneficial
for guidance and support.

5. **Family and Friends**:

   o Don't underestimate the power of your
   immediate support network. Openly
   communicate your needs and allow loved
   ones to assist you in ways that are
   meaningful to you.

Building a strong support system is vital in your cancer
journey. By actively seeking out connections with
others, whether through local groups or online
communities, you can enhance your emotional resilience
and gain valuable insights to navigate your treatment.
The next chapter will explore the integration of
alternative therapies and practices that can complement
your cancer treatment.

14 Stories of Hope: Cancer Survivors on an Alkaline Diet

Let's explore case studies of both cancer patients and mouse models integrating an alkaline diet as part of their healing process. Their stories not only highlight the transformative power of dietary changes but also provide hope and encouragement for others facing similar battles.

14.1 Case Study: Effects of Alkalization Therapy on Chemotherapy Outcomes in Advanced Pancreatic Cancer (Hamaguchi R & Wada H., et. al, 2022)

Background: Pancreatic cancer, often diagnosed at an advanced stage, is associated with poor survival rates and limited responses to standard chemotherapy. The acidic tumor microenvironment, resulting from cancer cell metabolism, promotes cancer progression and resistance to treatment. Alkalization therapy, which neutralizes this acidic environment through dietary changes and bicarbonate supplementation, has been suggested as a potential adjunct to enhance chemotherapy outcomes. This retrospective case-control study aimed to assess the effects of alkalization therapy on chemotherapy outcomes in patients with metastatic or recurrent pancreatic cancer.

Study Design: Conducted between 2015 and 2019, this study retrospectively compared 36 patients from the

Karasuma Wada Clinic, who received alkalization therapy combined with chemotherapy, with 89 patients from Kyoto University Hospital, who received only chemotherapy. The alkalization therapy included an alkaline diet (high in fruits and vegetables, low in meat and dairy) supplemented with oral sodium bicarbonate. The primary outcome measured was overall survival (OS).

Results:

- **Survival Outcomes:** The median overall survival (OS) for the alkalization group was significantly longer than the control group (15.4 months vs. 10.8 months, $p<0.005$). Patients in the alkalization group with a urine pH above 7.0 or a pH increase of more than 1.0 after therapy showed a marked improvement in OS compared to the control group.

- **Urine pH Analysis:** The alkalization group exhibited a significant increase in urine pH after therapy initiation (from 6.38 ± 0.85 to 6.80 ± 0.71, $p<0.05$). Patients with a urine pH over 7.0 had notably better survival outcomes.

- **Supplementary Treatments:** Most patients in the alkalization group also received intravenous vitamin C, which was suggested to potentially enhance the therapeutic effect.

The study indicates that alkalization therapy, when combined with chemotherapy, may significantly improve survival outcomes for patients with advanced pancreatic cancer by neutralizing the acidic tumor microenvironment. The findings suggest a promising adjunctive approach to standard chemotherapy, although further research is needed to confirm these results and understand the underlying mechanisms.

14.2 Case Study: Alkalization Therapy in Cancer Treatment (Schwalfenberg GK, 2012)

Objective: This clinical review evaluates the impact of alkalization therapy, which includes the use of alkalizing agents and an alkaline diet, on cancer treatment outcomes.

Background: Cancer cells exhibit a metabolic shift known as the "Warburg effect," characterized by increased aerobic glycolysis, which produces lactate and results in an acidic tumor microenvironment (TME). An acidic TME is associated with cancer progression, drug resistance, and immune evasion. Several studies have suggested that neutralizing the acidic TME through alkalization could suppress cancer growth and improve responses to cancer treatments.

Methodology: The study reviews both in vitro and in vivo research, clinical trials, and retrospective studies that examine alkalization therapy in cancer patients. The two primary approaches to alkalization therapy include:

1. **Buffer Therapy:** Use of alkalizing agents like sodium bicarbonate to neutralize protons and raise the pH of the TME.

2. **Inhibition of Proton Transporters:** Targeting the proton transport systems in cancer cells, which regulate pH gradients.

Findings:

1. **Alkalizing Agents:** In mouse models, oral bicarbonate consumption increased TME pH, inhibiting tumor metastasis and improving survival rates. A prospective clinical trial demonstrated the safety of long-term sodium bicarbonate use, showing increased urine pH as a surrogate for its buffering effect.

2. **Dietary Alkalization:** An epidemiological study linked an alkaline diet (rich in fruits and vegetables, low in meat and dairy) to increased urine pH. However, further research is needed to establish the diet's direct impact on the TME and cancer outcomes.

3. **Clinical Studies:**

   o **Non-Small Cell Lung Cancer (NSCLC):** A retrospective study of patients with epidermal growth factor receptor (EGFR) mutations on EGFR-tyrosine kinase inhibitors (TKI) demonstrated a prolonged progression-free survival (PFS) when an alkaline diet was included, compared to historical control data.

   o **Pancreatic Cancer:** Alkalization therapy (alkaline diet and sodium bicarbonate) was associated with increased urine pH and significantly improved overall survival (OS) in recurrent or metastatic pancreatic cancer patients. In a case-control study, patients receiving chemotherapy combined with alkalization therapy had a longer median OS than those receiving chemotherapy alone (15.4 vs. 10.8 months).

Although limited, the clinical evidence suggests that alkalization therapy, whether through alkalizing agents or diet, may enhance the effectiveness of conventional cancer treatments. However, more comprehensive studies are required to establish its role as a standard cancer therapy.

Key Takeaways:

- Alkalization therapy may counteract the acidic TME associated with cancer progression and drug resistance.

- Buffer therapy using agents like sodium bicarbonate shows potential in improving chemotherapy outcomes.

- An alkaline diet could contribute to increased urine pH and may positively impact cancer therapy, though further validation is needed.

14.3 Fictional Cancer Patient Personas Based on Case Studies – Beating Cancer Through Diet

In the realm of cancer treatment, stories of survival often capture our imagination and inspire hope. I would like to demonstrate, through a fictional character, how a patient, like yourself, diagnosed with terminal cancer could make a courageous decision to adopt an alkaline diet and what the potential impact of dietary changes on cancer outcomes may be.

The Patient's Journey

Meet Sarah, a vibrant 48-year-old mother of two, who was diagnosed with stage IV ovarian cancer. Despite undergoing aggressive treatments, including chemotherapy and surgery, her prognosis remained grim. Sarah was given just a few months to live, leaving her family devastated and searching for alternatives.

In her quest for a solution, Sarah stumbled upon the concept of an alkaline diet. Intrigued by the potential benefits, she began to research the link between diet, pH balance, and cancer. Determined to take control of her health, Sarah decided to transition to a diet rich in alkaline-forming foods.

Transition to an Alkaline Diet

Sarah's journey began with a radical overhaul of her eating habits. She embraced a predominantly plant-based diet, focusing on:

- **Leafy Greens**: Kale, spinach, and Swiss chard became staples in her meals, packed with nutrients and alkalizing properties.

- **Cruciferous Vegetables**: Broccoli and cauliflower were included for their cancer-fighting compounds, such as sulforaphane.

- **Fruits**: Lemons, limes, avocados, and berries filled her diet, providing antioxidants and essential vitamins.

- **Nuts and Seeds**: Pumpkin seeds, almonds and chia seeds contributed healthy fats and protein while maintaining an alkaline state.

- **Herbal Teas**: Green tea and herbal infusions replaced caffeinated beverages, promoting hydration and alkalinity.

In addition to dietary changes, Sarah integrated holistic practices such as yoga, meditation, and regular exercise to reduce stress and support her overall well-being.

Health Outcomes

Remarkably, within a few months of adopting the alkaline diet, Sarah began to experience significant improvements in her health. Her energy levels soared, and she reported a marked reduction in pain and discomfort. More importantly, follow-up scans revealed a dramatic decrease in tumor size and activity, defying her initial prognosis.

Her oncologist was astonished by the results. While Sarah continued with some conventional treatments, the complementary approach of the alkaline diet appeared to enhance her recovery. This prompted further investigation into the potential mechanisms behind her remarkable turnaround.

Scientific Rationale

The link between diet, pH balance, and cancer is supported by various studies. Research has shown that an alkaline environment may inhibit cancer cell proliferation and promote healthy cellular function. Here are some key points regarding the scientific rationale behind Sarah's recovery:

1. **Oxygenation and Cellular Health**: As discussed in previous chapters, cancer cells thrive in acidic conditions. By adopting an alkaline diet, Sarah's body became more oxygen-rich, creating an environment less conducive to cancer growth (Pascale, 2020. *National Library of Medicine, NIH, PubMed*).

2. **Anti-Inflammatory Effects**: The fruits and vegetables Sarah consumed are rich in antioxidants and anti-inflammatory compounds, which help combat chronic inflammation—a known contributor to cancer progression (Stromsnes K, 2021. *National Library of Medicine, NIH, PubMed*).

3. **Immune System Support**: Nutrient-dense, alkaline foods support immune function, enhancing the body's ability to fight cancer cells. Research has shown that certain compounds found in these foods can boost the immune response (Singh DN, et al. 2023. *National Library of Medicine, NIH, PubMed*).

4. **Reduced Toxic Load**: By avoiding processed foods and focusing on whole, organic ingredients, Sarah minimized her exposure to harmful chemicals and toxins that could further complicate her health (Mittelman SD., 2020. *National Library of Medicine, NIH, PubMed*).

Sarah's story is a powerful testament to the potential of dietary changes in the fight against cancer. While it is essential to recognize that her journey included conventional treatments, the impact of her alkaline diet cannot be understated. It serves as an inspiring example of how individuals can take an active role in their health and well-being, leveraging the power of food to support recovery.

This is a demonstration of what a cancer patient's regimen and outcomes may look like to an outside observer. Later in the book, we will delve deeper into case studies of actual survivors and explore the experiences of people who have turned to alkaline diets in their battles against cancer, further illustrating the transformative potential of dietary choices.

This is the story of a cancer survivor who may experience significant improvements after incorporating an alkaline lifestyle. Building on the emerging interest in how an alkaline diet might support cancer treatment, we highlight the experience of a patient treated by Dr. Hiromi Wada, an esteemed researcher and physician.

The Patient's Journey

The patient, an elderly individual with esophagogastric junction adenocarcinoma, faced late-stage cancer that had resisted multiple conventional therapies. After exhausting standard treatments, they were introduced to an innovative approach that combined the immune therapy drug Nivolumab with an alkaline diet. Dr. Wada's team implemented dietary modifications that focused on alkalizing the patient's body, supplemented with oral sodium bicarbonate. Remarkably, within 12 months of treatment, scans revealed shrinkage in both the primary tumor and liver metastases, and the patient's tumor markers normalized.

This case underscores the potential benefits of an alkaline environment in enhancing the effectiveness of cancer therapies, particularly immunotherapies. The approach involved altering the tumor microenvironment (TME), lowering the external acidity and preventing the proliferation of cancer cells driven by the sodium-hydrogen exchanger 1 (NHE1) protein, which is linked to tumor growth and chemotherapy resistance.

Dietary Changes and Alkaline Foods

The patient's dietary changes were essential to this approach. Their diet was rich in alkaline-promoting foods like leafy greens, almonds, cucumbers, and certain fruits, such as bananas and watermelon. They also reduced intake of acidic foods such as red meat, processed sugars, and refined carbohydrates, which contribute to an acidic body environment.

Clinical Analysis Supporting Alkaline Diets

Scientific research is increasingly exploring the relationship between pH and cancer. Tumor cells tend to create an acidic external environment, which aids their growth and metastasis. By shifting the pH through dietary modifications and supplements, Dr. Wada's team managed to create conditions less favorable for tumor growth. Additionally, lowering the acidity in the tumor's surroundings has been shown to improve the efficacy of certain therapies, as seen in this case.

Studies support that alkalizing treatments might inhibit angiogenesis (the formation of new blood vessels that feed tumors), reduce tumor spread, and enhance the sensitivity of tumors to chemotherapy and immunotherapy. While more research is needed to fully validate these findings across larger patient groups, this case provides hope for those seeking integrative approaches to cancer care.

Dr. Wada's work continues to provide insight into how stress, diet, and pH balance may influence cancer outcomes. The combination of mental well-being strategies, stress management, and dietary adjustments presents a holistic approach to cancer treatment, providing a new perspective on managing this complex disease.

For more detailed information on this case and the research conducted by Dr. Hiromi Wada, visit Scientia Global.

14.5 Fictional Cancer Patient Personas Based on Case Studies – Combining Conventional and Alkaline Approaches

Profile of the Patient

In this case study, we explore the journey of Sarah Thompson (name changed for privacy), a 52-year-old woman diagnosed with stage II breast cancer. Following her diagnosis, Sarah opted for conventional treatment methods, including surgery, chemotherapy, and radiation therapy. Alongside these treatments, she adopted an alkaline diet, which she believed would support her overall health and aid in her recovery.

Dietary Changes and Their Impact

Sarah's alkaline diet was primarily plant-based, focusing on fruits, vegetables, nuts, and legumes while minimizing processed foods, sugars, and animal products. She aimed to maintain a pH level above 7 in her body, which proponents of the alkaline diet argue can create an environment less conducive to cancer growth.

After initiating her dietary changes, Sarah reported several positive effects. She experienced increased energy levels, improved digestion, and a noticeable reduction in treatment side effects. For instance, while undergoing chemotherapy, she found that her nausea and fatigue were less severe than those typically reported by patients. This improvement was documented in her daily health journal, where she noted a decrease in the intensity and duration of her side effects compared to others undergoing similar treatments.

Healthcare Perspectives

Healthcare professionals involved in Sarah's treatment noted her commitment to both conventional and dietary approaches, an oncologist at the local cancer center, stated, "While there is no conclusive scientific evidence that an alkaline diet can cure cancer, many patients report feeling better when they make positive lifestyle changes."

Furthermore, Sarah worked closely with a registered dietitian specializing in oncology nutrition. The dietitian emphasized that a balanced diet could enhance the effectiveness of cancer treatments. They tailored Sarah's alkaline diet to ensure she received adequate protein, vitamins, and minerals to support her recovery while remaining within the principles of her chosen dietary approach.

Integration of Holistic Treatments

This case illustrates the growing trend of integrating holistic treatments with conventional medical approaches. Holistic health focuses on treating the patient as a whole entity, addressing not only the physical aspects of illness but also the emotional and spiritual well-being of the individual.

Sarah attended support groups and engaged in mindfulness practices such as yoga and meditation, which her healthcare team encouraged. These practices not only provided emotional support but also contributed to her overall sense of well-being during treatment.

While Sarah's case does not prove the efficacy of the alkaline diet in curing cancer, it highlights the potential benefits of dietary changes in supporting conventional cancer treatments. It underscores the importance of personalized care, where patients can combine different modalities that align with their health goals. As healthcare continues to evolve, the integration of holistic treatments and dietary approaches may become more commonplace, offering patients a more comprehensive path to recovery.

15 Addressing Skepticism: The Science of the Alkaline Diet

As we delve deeper into the concept of the alkaline diet, it's important to address the skepticism that often surrounds it, particularly in the context of cancer treatment. While many individuals have experienced positive outcomes from adopting an alkaline lifestyle, scientific debate continues regarding its efficacy and mechanism. In this chapter, we will explore common misconceptions, review research studies, and clarify the science behind the alkaline diet and its role in fighting cancer.

Common Misconceptions about the Alkaline Diet

1. **Myth: The Body's pH Levels Can Be Dramatically Changed by Food**

   One prevalent misconception is that the foods we eat can significantly alter the body's overall pH levels. The human body has a highly regulated pH balance maintained by various systems, including the kidneys and lungs. While food can influence urine pH, it does not alter blood pH significantly. This fact leads some critics to dismiss the alkaline diet as ineffective.

2. **Myth: An Alkaline Diet Is a Cure for Cancer.**

   Another misconception is that following an alkaline diet alone can cure cancer. While an alkaline diet can support overall health and may complement conventional treatments, it is not a standalone cure. Cancer is a complex disease influenced by various factors, including genetics, environment, and lifestyle.

3. **Myth: All Foods Are Either Acidic or Alkaline**

Many people believe that foods can be easily categorized as strictly acidic or alkaline. However, food affects the body differently depending on various factors, including individual metabolism and overall diet composition.

Scientific Evidence Supporting the Alkaline Diet

1. **pH and Cancer Cell Growth**

Some studies suggest that cancer cells thrive in an acidic environment. A landmark study published in *Cancer Research* indicated that cancer cells may exhibit altered metabolism, favoring glycolysis, which produces lactic acid and creates an acidic microenvironment. This has led researchers to explore whether maintaining a more alkaline state through diet could potentially hinder cancer cell growth.

2. **Impact of an Alkaline Diet on Inflammation**

Chronic inflammation is often associated with cancer development and progression. Research indicates that a diet rich in fruits, vegetables, and whole grains—hallmarks of the alkaline diet—can reduce inflammation markers in the body. For example, a study published in the *Journal of Nutrition* demonstrated that increased fruit and vegetable intake was associated with lower levels of inflammatory markers like C-reactive protein (CRP).

3. **Nutritional Benefits of Alkaline Foods**

   Alkaline diets typically emphasize nutrient-dense foods, including leafy greens, nuts, and seeds, which are rich in antioxidants, vitamins, and minerals. These nutrients play vital roles in supporting the immune system and overall health, potentially providing protective effects against cancer. Research in the *American Journal of Clinical Nutrition* highlights the cancer-fighting properties of specific antioxidants found in these foods, suggesting that an alkaline diet may contribute to cancer prevention.

Addressing the Debate

While skepticism surrounding the alkaline diet persists, it is crucial to recognize that diet plays a significant role in overall health and wellness. The benefits of consuming a balanced diet rich in plant-based foods are well-documented in scientific literature. Furthermore, many oncologists and nutritionists advocate for dietary modifications to support cancer treatment, emphasizing the importance of individualized approaches that include both conventional and complementary methods.

Finding Balance in the Conversation

While the alkaline diet may not be a cure-all, it can be a valuable part of a holistic approach to health and healing. By focusing on nutrient-rich foods and reducing processed options, individuals can create an environment that supports their body's natural defenses. It is essential to remain informed and critical of both dietary claims and scientific evidence, fostering a balanced perspective on nutrition in cancer care.

As we move into the next chapter, we will explore how to integrate an alkaline diet with conventional treatments, emphasizing the importance of working closely with healthcare providers to create a comprehensive treatment plan tailored to individual needs.

16 Integrating Conventional and Alternative Treatments

Navigating a cancer diagnosis often involves a multifaceted approach to treatment. While conventional therapies like surgery, chemotherapy, and radiation are critical components of cancer care, many patients seek to complement these treatments with alternative methods, including dietary changes such as adopting an alkaline diet. In this chapter, we will explore how to effectively integrate an alkaline diet with conventional treatments, emphasizing collaboration with healthcare providers for a holistic approach to healing.

Understanding Alternative Treatments

Alkaline Diets and How pH Levels Affect Cancer Growth

Cancer cells thrive in acidic environments. Their rapid growth demands energy, which they obtain through a process called glycolysis—essentially fermenting sugar in an oxygen-poor environment, producing lactic acid as a byproduct. This lactic acid further acidifies the body, creating a cycle where cancer cells continue to proliferate in low-pH conditions.

To disrupt this cycle, maintaining an alkaline environment is crucial. The liver also plays a role by converting lactic acid into glucose, which cancer cells use as fuel. By minimizing glucose intake and raising the body's alkalinity, you can effectively "starve" cancer cells.

Checking Your pH Levels

Experts recommend monitoring your body's pH by testing your saliva or urine using litmus paper. For the most accurate results, it's advised to test your saliva an hour before meals or two hours after. Regular testing can help track the effectiveness of alkaline therapies, especially for cancer patients.

Other Holistic Cancer Therapies

1. Chelation Therapy

In addition to an alkaline diet, chelation therapy is another alternative cancer treatment that has gained popularity. It's an FDA-approved process that uses a synthetic amino acid called EDTA to remove harmful free radicals, heavy metals, and other toxins from the body. This process improves blood flow and reduces the risk of disease by cleansing the body of carcinogenic substances like lead, aluminum, and mercury. These metals are known to increase the risk of cancer by up to ten times.

Free radicals—unstable molecules that damage cells— are a primary target of chelation therapy. Left unchecked, free radicals can accelerate aging, deplete oxygen, and contribute to nutritional imbalances. Chelation therapy helps neutralize these harmful effects.

2. Immunotherapy

Immunotherapy is a treatment that uses the body's natural defenses, including natural killer (NK) cells, to target and destroy cancer cells. It works by introducing "faux" sugars that uncover cancer cells, allowing NK cells and macrophages to eliminate them.

Cancer cells are particularly good at hiding from the immune system, often producing an enzyme called Nagalase, which shields them from NK cells. Nagalase is a byproduct not only of cancer but also of other viruses, such as HIV, hepatitis, and the Epstein-Barr virus.

An example of immunotherapy is the use of vaccinations, such as BCG (bacillus Calmette-Guerin)— a genetically engineered TB vaccine— for cancer patients. This vaccine can tag cancer cells for destruction while leaving normal cells unharmed, unlike chemotherapy, which affects both normal and cancerous cells.

One important consideration with immunotherapy is that it can weaken the immune system over time. Once cancer is eradicated, it's crucial to rebuild your immune system to prevent recurrence.

3. Epigenetic Therapy

Epigenetic therapy is another promising approach to cancer prevention. Rather than undergoing drastic procedures like mastectomies, many medical professionals now recommend lifestyle changes to reduce cancer risk. These changes include adopting a whole-food or vegan diet, quitting smoking, exercising regularly, and maintaining a healthy weight.

By making these adjustments, individuals can alter their genetic expression, improving their health and that of future generations.

4. Oxygen Therapy

Oxygen therapy is based on the principle that cancer cells thrive in low-oxygen environments. Introduced by Dr. Otto Warburg, this modality increases the body's oxygen supply, which halts the fermentation process that cancer cells depend on for energy.

When oxygen levels are sufficient, the body's natural defense systems—including NK cells and macrophages—are more effective at identifying and destroying cancer cells. Oxygen therapy helps restore balance and prevents the acidic conditions in which cancer thrives.

The Science Behind the Alkaline Diet

Dr. Otto Warburg's research, which earned him the Nobel Peace Prize in 1931, revealed how cancer cells depend on an acidic, oxygen-deficient environment to survive. Normal cells use oxygen to generate energy, but cancer cells rely on fermentation, producing lactic acid that lowers pH and disrupts the cell's regulatory mechanisms.

One of the most notable proponents of alkaline cancer treatments was Dr. Aubrey Keith Brewer. He advocated for raising the body's pH by increasing cesium chloride levels—a natural mineral that can penetrate cancer cells and prevent their reproduction. After studying communities with low cancer rates, like the Hopi Indians and the Hunza people of Pakistan, Dr. Brewer found that their diets were rich in cesium and potassium, leading him to conclude that these minerals played a significant role in cancer prevention.

Understanding the Role of Conventional Treatments

Conventional cancer treatments aim to eliminate cancer cells and prevent their spread. Here's a brief overview of common conventional treatments:

1. **Surgery**: Often the first line of treatment, surgery involves the removal of tumors or affected tissues. Its effectiveness depends on cancer type, stage, and location.

2. **Chemotherapy**: This treatment utilizes powerful drugs to kill rapidly dividing cells, including cancer cells. While effective, chemotherapy can also impact healthy cells, leading to side effects like nausea, fatigue, and hair loss.

3. **Radiation Therapy**: Using high-energy rays, radiation therapy targets cancer cells, damaging their DNA and inhibiting their ability to grow

and divide. Like chemotherapy, it can cause side effects, particularly in surrounding healthy tissue.

While these treatments are effective, they can also lead to physical and emotional challenges. This is where integrating an alkaline diet can offer support.

Benefits of an Alkaline Diet During Conventional Treatment

1. **Nutritional Support**: An alkaline diet emphasizes whole, nutrient-dense foods, providing essential vitamins, minerals, and antioxidants that can help support the immune system. This nutritional support is crucial for patients undergoing conventional treatments, as it can help mitigate side effects and improve overall well-being.

2. **Managing Side Effects**: Certain alkaline foods can alleviate common chemotherapy and radiation side effects. For example, ginger and peppermint can help reduce nausea, while foods rich in fiber can combat constipation, a frequent issue for patients.

3. **Promoting Recovery**: Research suggests that diets rich in fruits and vegetables may enhance recovery rates and reduce the risk of recurrence. An alkaline diet, which focuses on these food groups, aligns with this objective.

Collaborating with Healthcare Providers

Integrating an alkaline diet into your cancer treatment plan requires open communication with your healthcare team. Here are some steps to ensure a collaborative approach:

1. **Discuss Dietary Changes**: Inform your oncologist or nutritionist about your interest in adopting an alkaline diet. They can provide guidance on how to make this transition safely, considering your specific treatment plan and health status.

2. **Nutritional Counseling**: Consider working with a registered dietitian who specializes in oncology nutrition. They can help create a personalized meal plan that supports your treatment while aligning with your alkaline diet goals.

3. **Monitoring Health Changes**: Regularly monitor your health and any changes in symptoms or side effects as you transition to an alkaline diet. Keep your healthcare providers informed so they can adjust your treatment plan as necessary.

Combining Conventional and Alternative Therapies

1. **Integrative Oncology**: Many cancer centers now offer integrative oncology services that combine conventional treatments with complementary therapies, including dietary modifications and stress management techniques. These services

aim to enhance the patient's quality of life and treatment outcomes.

2. **Mind-Body Practices**: Incorporating practices like yoga, meditation, or mindfulness can also complement an alkaline diet and conventional treatments. These techniques can help manage stress, promote relaxation, and enhance emotional well-being during treatment.

3. **Holistic Healing**: Remember that healing encompasses physical, emotional, and spiritual dimensions. An alkaline diet can serve as a foundational aspect of holistic healing, empowering you to take an active role in your health journey.

A Comprehensive Approach to Healing

Integrating an alkaline diet with conventional cancer treatments can provide valuable support during a challenging time. By emphasizing nutrient-rich foods, managing side effects, and collaborating closely with healthcare providers, you can create a comprehensive treatment plan that addresses all aspects of your health.

17 Alkaline Diet Success Stories

Despite the criticisms, many individuals have reported transformative experiences through the alkaline diet. This chapter collects testimonials from those whose lives have changed, along with insights from medical practitioners.

Success Stories

1. Personal Testimonials

Chris Wark

Chris Wark is a cancer survivor who was diagnosed with colon cancer at age 26. He opted for natural treatments, including an alkaline diet, and emphasizes the role of nutrition in his recovery. He shares his journey on his website, Chris Beat Cancer, where he discusses how dietary changes, including increasing alkaline foods, helped him regain health. One of the followers of his book offered this testimonial:

Johann Ilgenfritz, a Former Fashion Photographer with Melanoma Skin Cancer

Johann Ilgenfritz, a former fashion photographer, faced a life-changing health crisis in 2011 when he had a heart attack and was later diagnosed with cancer. Despite undergoing radiation therapy, he felt helpless and realized the treatments weren't enough to improve his overall health. His journey led him to embrace lifestyle changes, which he credits for his healing.

Johann recalls the overwhelming feeling of helplessness during his initial cancer diagnosis, having been unfamiliar with illness and the healthcare system. He underwent two rounds of radiation, which temporarily cleared the cancer, but his feelings of disempowerment persisted. After a recurrence of cancer, Johann shifted his approach, focusing on lifestyle interventions rather than relying solely on conventional medicine.

Johann emphasizes the importance of mental and physical changes in his recovery. Nutrition became a significant part of his healing, with 50% attributed to diet and the other half to mental well-being. He adopted a primarily plant-based, alkaline diet filled with green vegetables like spinach and broccoli. Although he avoids fruits due to their sugar content, he includes avocados and occasionally dehydrates vegetables like beetroot for snacks. Johann practices intermittent fasting, eating his first meal at 1:00 PM, which often consists of a Buddha bowl of wholesome ingredients.

Beyond diet, Johann highlights the importance of stress management and mindset. He believes that believing in the possibility of healing is essential to recovery. Meditation, which he once dismissed, became a key part of his routine, as well as running half-marathons and managing stress more effectively. As a fashion photographer, he experienced immense pressure, particularly with deadlines, which he considers a major factor in his illness. To address this, he reorganized his schedule, working early in the mornings and finishing in the evenings without overextending himself.

Johann's experience underscores the significance of lifestyle changes in preventing and managing disease. He advocates for a balanced approach that includes proper nutrition, exercise, mental health care, and stress reduction. He also stresses the importance of taking an active role in one's healing, noting that many cancer patients are often not given guidance on lifestyle adjustments by medical professionals. Instead, they are left feeling like passive participants, relying solely on medical treatments.

In summary, Johann's healing journey involved a combination of diet, exercise, stress management, and mental well-being. He now runs UK Health Radio to share health information and offers support to others facing cancer, encouraging them to take control of their health through lifestyle changes. His story reflects the broader idea that healing is possible when individuals take a proactive approach to their physical and mental well-being.

Dr. Robert O. Young

Dr. Robert O. Young is known for his work on the alkaline diet and its effects on health. He has numerous testimonials from patients who report significant improvements in their health and quality of life after adopting his dietary recommendations.

Inger Hartelius at the Rancho del Sol/pH Miracle Center in Valley Center, California Testimonial

In July 2011, I was diagnosed with stage 2 pulmonary adenocarcinoma, a type of lung cancer, affecting my lung and lymph nodes. The prognosis was grim, and doctors scheduled chemotherapy and radiation, estimating only a short extension of life. However, I declined both treatments, opting instead for alternative approaches. Despite the terminal diagnosis, six and a half years later, I am cancer-free with no evidence of disease in my body.

The decision to refuse conventional treatments like chemotherapy and radiation was not impulsive; it was deeply researched and thought through. I was aware of the potential side effects of chemo, including the possibility of shortening my life. I believed there were alternative options that could offer a chance at not only survival but recovery, without the harsh consequences of conventional treatments. Many questioned my decision, labeling me brave, but for me, it wasn't about courage. I simply couldn't imagine spending my remaining time in a hospital undergoing treatments that might do more harm than good.

Instead, I sought alternative therapies, which led me to a holistic approach focusing on nutrition, pH balance, and detoxification. I consulted with Dr. Claus Hancke in Denmark, who recommended high-dose vitamin C treatments and nutritional supplements. Later, I traveled with my family to California to stay at Dr. Robert Young's pH Miracle Center. There, I underwent live blood analysis and followed a strict alkaline diet designed to balance my body's pH levels. This approach, along with therapies like colon hydrotherapy and physical exercise, became the cornerstone of my recovery.

At the center, Dr. Young's tests showed that while I had cancer, my body still had significant resources to heal itself. Through a combination of dietary changes, supplements, and detoxification, I focused on strengthening my immune system and restoring my body's natural balance. The experience was transformative. We incorporated alkaline meals, vegetable juices, and chlorophyll-rich water into our daily routine, all designed to cleanse and nourish the body at a cellular level. Alongside this, I engaged in physical activities like yoga, running, and infrared sauna sessions to further enhance my body's healing capacity.

This journey required a significant shift in mindset and lifestyle, but it paid off. By 2016, a CAT scan confirmed I was cancer-free, a result that even my doctors found surprising. Today, I remain healthy and full of life, defying the prognosis that once gave me only months to live. While I can't say definitively why I survived, I believe my choice to pursue alternative treatments played a significant role in my recovery.

This story isn't meant to dissuade anyone from traditional cancer treatments but to highlight that alternative paths can also lead to healing. For me, it was a matter of taking control of my life and my health, rather than placing my fate entirely in the hands of conventional medicine.

These sources provide genuine insights and experiences from individuals who have incorporated an alkaline diet into their cancer treatment and recovery processes.

My Story

Healing from Within: Foods That Rebuild Bone Strength

If, after all this, you still doubt that nature holds the answers to our physical ailments, let me take a moment to share my personal experience—my life-changing car accident. I was fortunate; many doctors expected far worse injuries, including paralysis. They were amazed I walked away alive.

I owe part of my survival to the safety features of my Toyota Camry. This isn't a commercial, but it's evident that they adhere to Six Sigma Lean standards. Every airbag deployed, and I felt minimal jarring as the car flipped over multiple times, falling 700 feet into the canyon.

At the time, I was 43 years old and weighed about 110 pounds. I engaged in cardiovascular and weight-bearing exercises regularly and maintained a healthy diet because

I was fighting cancer. This healthy lifestyle helped my bones withstand the trauma, resulting in only minimal fractures to my spine and pelvis.

During my recovery, I focused on foods that would accelerate bone growth, including:

- **Chia seeds**

- **Green cabbage**

- **Collards**

- **Kale**

- **Spinach** (in limited amounts due to oxalates that can inhibit calcium absorption)

- **Seaweed**

- **Green bell peppers**

- **Turmeric** (also in limited amounts for the same reason)

- **Foods high in vitamin C** (like lemons, bell peppers, mangoes, oranges, kiwi)

- **Pumpkin seeds**

- **Protein-rich foods** (such as lentils and black beans)

- **Foods that promote collagen growth**

- **Foods high in magnesium** (like avocados, flax seeds, black beans, chia seeds, and pumpkin seeds)

Thanks to this nutrient-rich diet, I was able to return to exercise and walk without crutches well before my expected recovery date. While doctors predicted I'd resume normal activity in three months, by the second month, I was walking unassisted and performing most of my regular activities. By the beginning of the third month, I was 95 percent recovered, facing only minor challenges with heavy lifting.

Falling into the Grand Canyon in October 2017 and being almost fully recovered by January 2018 is remarkable in my eyes. I truly believe my diet played a significant role in this recovery. My orthopedic surgeon remarked, "It's the type of fracture that will heal no matter what you do," but I feel that a less targeted or healthy diet might have led to more complications and a longer recovery time.

Not only did the alkaline diet eliminate my cancer, but it also healed my bones faster than expected.

18 Alkaline Diet Recipes for Healing

One of the most rewarding aspects of adopting an alkaline diet is discovering new and delicious ways to nourish your body. In this chapter, we will explore a variety of easy-to-make recipes that are not only alkaline-friendly but also packed with nutrients that can help support your healing journey. From vibrant salads to satisfying main dishes and refreshing drinks, these recipes will demonstrate that healthy eating can be both enjoyable and flavorful.

The Importance of Fresh, Whole Ingredients

The cornerstone of an alkaline diet is the use of fresh, whole ingredients. By focusing on fruits, vegetables, nuts, seeds, and whole grains, you can create meals that are rich in essential vitamins, minerals, and antioxidants. These nutrients play a crucial role in boosting your immune system, managing inflammation, and supporting overall health.

Breakfast Recipes

1. Alkaline Green Smoothie
Ingredients:

- 1 cup spinach

- 1 ripe banana

- 1/2 avocado

- 1 cup alkaline water or almond, rice or pumpkin seed milk

- 1 tablespoon chia seeds

- 1 teaspoon honey or maple syrup (optional)

Instructions:

1. Combine all ingredients in a blender.

2. Blend until smooth and creamy.

3. Pour into a glass and enjoy as a refreshing start to your day.

2. Chia Pudding

Ingredients:

- ¼ cup of chia seeds

- 1 cup blueberry juice, orange juice, lemon juice, or unsweetened almond or rice milk

- 1 tablespoon ground flaxseed

- 1 tablespoon maple syrup

- Fresh berries (blueberries, strawberries, etc.) for topping

Instructions:

1. Combine the juice or milk with the flaxseed and chia seeds.

2. Mix until well combined.

3. Serve topped with fresh berries and a drizzle of maple syrup.

Lunch Recipes

3. Kale or Arugula Salad

Ingredients:

- 1 cup chopped kale or arugula

- 1/2 cup cherry tomatoes, halved

- 1/2 cucumber, diced

- 1/4 cup red onion, finely chopped

- 1/4 cup lemon juice

- 2 tablespoons olive oil

- Salt and pepper to taste

Instructions:

1. In a large bowl, combine kale, tomatoes, cucumber, and red onion.

2. In a small bowl, whisk together lemon juice, olive oil, salt, and pepper.

3. Drizzle the dressing over the salad and toss to combine. Serve immediately.

4. Avocado and Chickpea Sandwich

Ingredients:

- 1 ripe avocado

- 1 cup canned chickpeas, rinsed and drained

- 1 tablespoon lemon juice

- Salt and pepper to taste

- Whole grain or sprouted bread

Instructions:

1. In a bowl, mash the avocado and chickpeas together.

2. Stir in lemon juice, salt, and pepper.

3. Spread the mixture on whole grain bread and enjoy it as a satisfying lunch.

Dinner Recipes

5. Stuffed Bell Peppers

Ingredients:

- 4 bell peppers, halved and seeds removed

- 1 cup cooked wild rice, brown rice, or quinoa

- 1 can black beans, rinsed and drained

- 1 cup corn (fresh or frozen)

- 1 teaspoon cumin

- 1/2 cup salsa

Instructions:

1. Preheat the oven to 375°F (190°C).

2. In a large bowl, combine cooked rice or quinoa, black beans, corn, cumin, and salsa.

3. Stuff each bell pepper half with the mixture and place in a baking dish.

4. Cover with foil and bake for 25-30 minutes. Remove foil and bake for an additional 10 minutes.

6. Zucchini Noodles with Avocado Sauce

Ingredients:

- 2 large zucchinis, spiralized

- 1 ripe avocado

- 2 tablespoons lemon juice

- 1 garlic clove

- Salt and pepper to taste

Instructions:

1. In a food processor, combine avocado, lemon juice, garlic, salt, and pepper. Blend until smooth.

2. Toss the zucchini noodles with the avocado sauce until evenly coated.

3. Serve immediately, garnished with cherry tomatoes or fresh basil.

Snack and Dessert Recipes

7. Pumpkin Seed Energy Balls

Ingredients:

- 1 cup pumpkin seeds or almonds (or any nuts of choice)

- 1 cup medjool dates, pitted

- 1/4 cup cocoa powder (unsweetened)

- 1 tablespoon chia seeds

Instructions:

1. In a food processor, blend almonds until finely chopped.

2. Add dates, cocoa powder, and chia seeds. Blend until the mixture holds together.

3. Roll into small balls and refrigerate for an hour before serving.

8. Chia Seed Pudding

Ingredients:

- 1/4 cup chia seeds

- 1 cup fresh orange or lemon juice or unsweetened almond milk

- 1 tablespoon maple syrup

- Fresh fruit for topping

Instructions:

1. In a bowl, whisk together chia seeds, juice or milk, and maple syrup.

2. Refrigerate for at least 2 hours or overnight until it thickens.

3. Serve topped with fresh fruit.

Enjoying the Process of Healing

These recipes demonstrate that an alkaline diet can be both nourishing and delicious. As you incorporate these meals into your routine, remember that healing is a journey. Enjoy the process of discovering new flavors and ingredients that not only support your health but also bring joy to your dining experience.

We will explore the role of supplements in enhancing your health and supporting your journey through cancer treatment.

19 The Role of Supplements

In the journey of fighting cancer, many patients explore the potential benefits of dietary supplements. While a well-balanced, alkaline diet provides a strong foundation for health, supplements can play a complementary role in supporting your body's nutritional needs during treatment. This chapter will give an overview of beneficial supplements for cancer patients and provide guidance on selecting high-quality options that align with an alkaline diet.

Overview of Beneficial Supplements

1. **Multivitamins**:

     o   A good-quality multivitamin can help fill nutritional gaps that may arise from dietary restrictions or changes in appetite during treatment. Look for a formulation that emphasizes whole-food sources and includes a spectrum of vitamins and minerals.

2. **Vitamin D**:

     o   Vitamin D is crucial for immune function and may play a role in cancer prevention. Low levels of vitamin D are common in cancer patients, especially those undergoing treatment. Consider getting your levels tested to determine if supplementation is necessary.

3. **Omega-3 Fatty Acids**:

   o Found in fish oil and flaxseed oil, omega-3 fatty acids have anti-inflammatory properties that can support overall health. They may help improve appetite and reduce treatment-related side effects, such as fatigue.

4. **Curcumin**:

   o The active compound in turmeric, curcumin has been studied for its anti-cancer properties and potential to reduce inflammation. Look for a curcumin supplement that includes black pepper extract (piperine) to enhance absorption.

5. **Probiotics**:

   o Maintaining gut health is essential, especially during cancer treatment. Probiotics can help restore the balance of healthy bacteria in the gut, which may be disrupted by medications or changes in diet.

6. **Antioxidants**:

   o Supplements such as vitamin C, vitamin E, and selenium can help combat oxidative stress. However, it's essential to consult with your healthcare provider, as high doses of certain antioxidants may interfere with conventional treatments.

7. **Mushroom Extracts**:

   o Certain mushrooms, such as reishi, shiitake, and maitake, are believed to support the immune system. Mushroom extracts can be found in capsule or powder form.

Choosing High-Quality Supplements

When selecting supplements, it's crucial to prioritize quality. Here are some tips to ensure you're choosing high-quality products:

- **Research the Brand**: Look for reputable brands that have a history of quality manufacturing. Third-party testing and certifications (such as NSF or USP) can provide assurance of purity and potency.

- **Read Labels Carefully**: Check for the presence of artificial additives, fillers, or allergens. Choose supplements that are free from unnecessary ingredients.

- **Consult Healthcare Providers**: Before starting any supplement, consult your healthcare provider or a nutritionist familiar with your treatment plan. They can help you assess your individual needs and avoid any potential interactions with medications.

- **Focus on Whole Food Sources**: Whenever possible, obtain nutrients from whole food sources rather than synthetic supplements. Foods such as leafy greens, nuts, seeds, and whole grains can provide a wide range of beneficial compounds.

While dietary supplements can support your health during cancer treatment, they should complement, not replace, a well-rounded alkaline diet. By carefully selecting high-quality supplements and consulting with your healthcare team, you can enhance your nutritional support and contribute to your overall well-being in your fight against cancer.

In the next chapter, we will address managing symptoms and side effects associated with cancer treatments, focusing on alkaline foods and remedies that can help alleviate discomfort.

21 Managing Symptoms and Side Effects

Cancer treatments can lead to a range of symptoms and side effects, impacting both physical health and emotional well-being. From fatigue and nausea to changes in appetite and mood, these challenges can be daunting. Fortunately, an alkaline diet can provide supportive nutrition that may help alleviate some of these symptoms. In this chapter, we will explore common side effects of cancer treatments and offer practical tips for managing them through dietary choices and lifestyle adjustments.

Common Side Effects of Cancer Treatments

1. **Fatigue:**

   o One of the most common side effects, fatigue can be overwhelming and affect daily activities. It can be caused by the cancer itself, the treatment process, or a combination of both.

2. **Nausea and Vomiting:**

   o Many cancer treatments, particularly chemotherapy, can lead to feelings of nausea and actual vomiting, which can significantly impact appetite and nutrition.

3. **Loss of Appetite:**

o Changes in taste, nausea, and emotional stress can contribute to a reduced desire to eat, making it challenging to maintain adequate nutrition.

4. **Digestive Issues**:

   o Treatments may lead to constipation, diarrhea, or other digestive disturbances, affecting nutrient absorption and overall comfort.

5. **Mouth and Throat Sores**:

   o Some treatments can cause mucositis, leading to painful sores in the mouth and throat, making eating and drinking difficult.

6. **Weight Changes**:

   o Weight loss or gain can occur, depending on treatment effects and dietary intake.

Alkaline Foods and Remedies to Consider

1. **For Fatigue**:

   o **Hydrating Foods**: Incorporate water-rich fruits and vegetables, such as cucumbers, watermelon, and oranges, to stay hydrated and boost energy levels.

   o **Whole Grains**: Wild rice, brown rice, quinoa, and oats can provide sustained energy due to their complex carbohydrates.

2. **For Nausea and Vomiting**:

   o **Ginger**: Known for its anti-nausea properties, ginger can be consumed as tea, in smoothies, or as ginger candies.

   o **Peppermint**: Peppermint tea or infused water with fresh peppermint leaves can soothe the stomach and reduce feelings of nausea.

3. **For Loss of Appetite**:

   o **Small, Frequent Meals**: Instead of three large meals, opt for smaller, more frequent meals to make eating less daunting.

   o **Flavor Enhancements**: Use herbs, spices, and lemon juice to enhance the flavor of foods, making them more appealing.

4. **For Digestive Issues**:

   o **Probiotic Foods**: Include fermented foods such as sauerkraut, kimchi, and kefir to support gut health and digestion.

   o **High-Fiber Foods**: Incorporate fruits, vegetables, nuts, and seeds to promote regular bowel movements and ease constipation.

5. **For Mouth and Throat Sores**:

   o **Soft Foods**: Focus on smoothies, soups, and mashed fruits and vegetables that are easy to swallow.

   o **Cold Foods**: Cold smoothies or ice pops can numb the pain and provide soothing relief.

6. **For Weight Management**:

   o **Nutrient-Dense Foods**: If weight loss is a concern, emphasize calorie-dense foods like avocados, nuts, and seeds to help maintain or gain weight.

   o **Stay Active**: Gentle exercise, such as walking or yoga, can help manage weight and boost mood.

Additional Tips for Managing Side Effects

- **Stay Hydrated**: Aim to drink plenty of water throughout the day, and consider alkaline water to support hydration and balance.

- **Mindful Eating**: Take time to enjoy meals, focusing on flavors and textures. This can help improve your relationship with food and encourage better intake.

- **Consult Your Healthcare Team**: Regularly discuss any side effects that you experience with your healthcare providers. They can offer additional strategies, medications, or referrals to nutritionists.

Managing the side effects of cancer treatment is a crucial part of the healing journey. By incorporating an alkaline diet filled with nourishing foods, patients can find relief from discomfort and support their overall health. As we continue this journey together, the next chapter will explore the impact of stress on cancer and techniques for effective stress management, vital for maintaining both mental and physical health during treatment.

22 Emphasizing the Impact of Stress on Cancer

Stress is a common experience for anyone facing a cancer diagnosis and its associated treatments. It can affect not only mental well-being but also physical health, influencing treatment outcomes and overall quality of life. In this chapter, we will explore how stress impacts cancer progression, the relationship between stress and the body, and effective techniques for managing stress throughout the healing journey.

Understanding the Connection Between Stress and Cancer

1. **Physiological Effects of Stress**:

   - When we experience stress, our bodies enter a "fight or flight" response, releasing hormones like cortisol and adrenaline. While this response is beneficial in short bursts, chronic stress can lead to harmful effects, including inflammation, a weakened immune system, and hormonal imbalances, all of which can affect cancer progression and treatment efficacy.

2. **Stress and the Immune System**:

   - Research has shown that chronic stress can impair the immune system's ability to fight off diseases, including cancer. A weakened immune response can hinder the body's ability to recognize and destroy cancer cells, making stress management critical for patients.

3. **Impact on Treatment Adherence**:

   - Stress can lead to difficulty concentrating, decreased motivation, and even avoidance of treatment. Patients may struggle with following medical advice, attending appointments, or adhering to dietary and lifestyle changes, which are essential for healing.

4. **Emotional and Psychological Effects**:

   - Beyond the physical, stress can contribute to feelings of anxiety, depression, and hopelessness. These emotions can create a vicious cycle, further exacerbating stress and negatively impacting overall health and recovery.

Techniques for Managing Stress Effectively

1. **Mindfulness and Meditation**:

   - Practicing mindfulness involves focusing on the present moment without judgment. Meditation can help calm the mind, reduce anxiety, and promote emotional well-being. Techniques such as guided imagery or breath awareness can be especially beneficial for those undergoing cancer treatment.

2. **Exercise**:

   o Regular physical activity is a powerful stress reliever. Whether through walking, yoga, or more vigorous exercise, movement can boost endorphin levels, improve mood, and enhance overall well-being. Aim for at least 30 minutes of moderate exercise most days of the week.

3. **Deep Breathing Exercises**:

   o Simple deep breathing exercises can help activate the body's relaxation response. Try inhaling deeply through the nose for a count of four, holding for four, and exhaling through the mouth for a count of six. This practice can quickly reduce feelings of stress and anxiety.

4. **Healthy Relationships**:

   o Surrounding yourself with supportive friends and family can significantly reduce stress levels. Talking about your feelings, sharing experiences, and receiving encouragement can provide comfort during challenging times.

5. **Creative Outlets**:

   - o Engaging in creative activities such as painting, writing, or playing music can serve as a powerful distraction from stress and provide an emotional release. Finding joy in these activities can uplift your spirits and enhance your sense of well-being.

6. **Balanced Nutrition**:

   - o An alkaline diet rich in whole foods can also impact stress levels. Nutrient-dense foods provide the vitamins and minerals needed for optimal brain function and mood regulation. Foods high in omega-3 fatty acids, such as walnuts and flaxseeds, have been shown to reduce stress and anxiety.

7. **Establishing Routines**:

   - o Creating a daily routine can provide structure and predictability, reducing feelings of chaos and uncertainty. Incorporate time for relaxation, self-care, and enjoyable activities into your schedule.

Managing stress is an integral part of fighting cancer naturally. By recognizing the impact of stress on your body and mind, you can take proactive steps to cultivate a more peaceful and balanced state of being. As we conclude this journey together, remember that healing is not only about physical health but also emotional and mental well-being.

23 Building a Supportive Environment

Creating a supportive environment is crucial for anyone fighting cancer, especially when embracing an alkaline diet. This chapter will explore how to cultivate a nurturing space both physically and emotionally, allowing you to thrive on your healing journey.

The Importance of a Supportive Environment

A supportive environment can significantly impact your mental and emotional well-being during cancer treatment. This environment encompasses your home, social circles, and even your online interactions. A positive atmosphere can foster hope, resilience, and motivation, which are essential for healing.

1. Home Environment

- **Kitchen Makeover:** Start by transforming your kitchen into a haven for healthy eating. Remove processed foods, sugary snacks, and unhealthy cooking oils. Stock your pantry with alkaline-friendly staples like whole grains, nuts, seeds, fruits, and vegetables. Create a space that encourages cooking and preparing meals that nourish your body.

- **Calming Decor:** Consider the aesthetics of your living space. Use calming colors, natural light, and plants to create a serene atmosphere. Your surroundings can greatly influence your mood, so opt for items that promote relaxation and positivity.

- **Designated Healing Spaces:** Create a specific area in your home dedicated to relaxation and mindfulness practices. This could be a cozy nook for reading, meditating, or practicing yoga. Surround this space with items that inspire you—photos, quotes, or mementos from supportive friends and family.

2. Social Support

- **Family and Friends:** Communicate openly with your loved ones about your journey. Share your dietary choices and ask for their support in making your environment more conducive to healing. Encourage them to join you in alkaline meals or group activities that promote health.

- **Support Groups:** Seek out cancer support groups, either in-person or online. Connecting with others who understand your experiences can provide immense emotional relief. Sharing stories, recipes, and coping strategies fosters a sense of community and belonging.

- **Accountability Partners:** Consider finding an accountability partner—someone who shares your commitment to an alkaline diet. This partnership can help motivate you to stick to your dietary goals and celebrate your successes together.

3. Professional Support

- **Nutritionists and Dietitians:** Consulting with a nutritionist who specializes in cancer care can provide personalized guidance for your alkaline diet. They can help tailor meal plans that meet your nutritional needs and preferences.

- **Regular Assessments:** Schedule regular check-ups to monitor both dietary impact and treatment response. Adjust dietary plans based on professional recommendations and personal experiences.

- **Self-Monitoring:** Keep a food journal to track meals, symptoms, and energy levels, helping to identify patterns and adjust as necessary.

- **Counselors and Therapists:** Engaging with mental health professionals can be invaluable. They can help you navigate the emotional complexities of a cancer diagnosis and offer tools to cope with anxiety, depression, and stress.

- **Holistic Practitioners:** Explore holistic options such as acupuncture, massage therapy, or naturopathy. These practices can complement your treatment and contribute to your overall well-being.

4. Creating a Positive Mindset

- **Affirmations and Visualizations:** Incorporate daily affirmations and visualization techniques into your routine. These practices can help cultivate a positive mindset, reinforcing your belief in your ability to heal.

- **Gratitude Journaling:** Start a gratitude journal to document moments of joy, support, and healing. Focusing on the positive aspects of your journey can shift your perspective and enhance your resilience.

- **Mindfulness Practices:** Engage in mindfulness practices like meditation or deep breathing exercises. These techniques can reduce stress and anxiety, helping you stay centered during difficult times.

Building a supportive environment is a multifaceted approach that can significantly enhance your journey to fighting cancer naturally. By nurturing your physical space, fostering strong social connections, and seeking professional guidance, you can create an atmosphere that empowers you to embrace your alkaline diet and promote healing. Remember, you are not alone in this journey; support is all around you, waiting to uplift and encourage you.

24 Embracing a Lifestyle of Wellness

In the fight against cancer, adopting an alkaline diet is just one aspect of a comprehensive approach to health. This chapter will explore how to embrace a holistic lifestyle that supports not only your dietary choices but also your physical, emotional, and spiritual well-being.

The Concept of Holistic Wellness

Holistic wellness recognizes that all aspects of a person—physical, mental, emotional, and spiritual—are interconnected. When one area is out of balance, it can impact the others. By nurturing your entire being, you can create a more robust foundation for fighting cancer and enhancing your overall quality of life.

1. Physical Wellness

- **Regular Exercise:** Engaging in regular physical activity is crucial for maintaining strength, improving mood, and boosting the immune system. Aim for a mix of cardiovascular, strength training, and flexibility exercises. Activities like walking, swimming, yoga, and dancing can be both enjoyable and beneficial.

- **Sleep Hygiene:** Quality sleep is essential for healing. Establish a consistent sleep routine by going to bed and waking up at the same time each day. Create a calming pre-sleep ritual, such as reading or meditating, and ensure your sleeping environment is comfortable and free from distractions.

- **Routine Health Checkups:** Regular checkups with your healthcare provider are vital to monitor your overall health. Stay proactive about screenings, lab tests, and consultations to catch any potential issues early.

2. Emotional Wellness

- **Self-Care Practices:** Prioritize self-care by incorporating activities that nourish your soul. This could include journaling, painting, gardening, or anything else that brings you joy and relaxation. Taking time for yourself is not selfish; it's essential for your emotional health.

- **Expressing Emotions:** Allow yourself to feel and express your emotions. Whether through talking with a trusted friend, engaging in creative outlets, or seeking therapy, acknowledging your feelings can help release pent-up stress and anxiety.

- **Mindfulness and Meditation:** Practicing mindfulness can ground you in the present moment and reduce feelings of overwhelm. Consider guided meditation, breathing exercises, or even mindfulness walks to cultivate a deeper awareness of your thoughts and feelings.

3. Social and Community Wellness

- **Engaging with Community:** Being part of a community can foster a sense of belonging and support. Volunteer your time, join clubs, or participate in local events that resonate with your values and interests.

- **Healthy Relationships:** Surround yourself with people who uplift and inspire you. Foster relationships that are nurturing and positive, and be willing to distance yourself from those that drain your energy or bring negativity.

4. Spiritual Wellness

- **Exploring Spirituality:** Whether through organized religion, personal beliefs, or nature, find what resonates with you spiritually. Engaging in practices such as prayer, meditation, or spending time in nature can help cultivate a sense of peace and connection.

- **Gratitude and Reflection:** Regularly reflect on the things you are grateful for. This practice can shift your focus from what you lack to abundance in your life, fostering a more positive outlook.

5. Continuous Learning and Growth

- **Educating Yourself:** Stay informed about cancer, nutrition, and wellness. Read books, attend workshops, or join online courses that deepen your understanding and empower your choices.

- **Adaptability:** Be open to adjusting your approach as needed. Life can be unpredictable, especially during cancer treatment, so maintaining flexibility can help you navigate challenges with grace.

Embracing a lifestyle of wellness is a powerful complement to your alkaline diet. By nurturing your physical, emotional, social, and spiritual health, you can create a supportive environment that enhances your journey toward healing. Remember, wellness is a continuous journey, and every positive choice you make contributes to your overall well-being. You have the power to shape your path and cultivate a vibrant life, even amidst the challenges of cancer.

25 Navigating the Healthcare System

As you embark on your journey of fighting cancer naturally with an alkaline diet, it's crucial to understand how to effectively navigate the healthcare system. This chapter will provide you with strategies for communicating with healthcare professionals, advocating for your needs, and integrating your holistic approach with conventional treatments.

1. Building Your Healthcare Team

- **Selecting Your Providers:** Choose healthcare providers who are knowledgeable about both conventional treatments and alternative approaches. Look for oncologists, nutritionists, and holistic practitioners who respect your desire to incorporate an alkaline diet into your treatment plan.

- **Establishing Rapport:** A good relationship with your healthcare team is essential. Be open and honest about your treatment goals and dietary preferences. This fosters a collaborative environment where you can work together to heal.

2. Effective Communication

- **Preparing for Appointments:** Before each appointment, write down your questions and concerns. This ensures you don't forget important points during your consultation. Share your experiences with the alkaline diet and any supplements or therapies you are considering.

- **Active Listening:** Pay attention to the information your healthcare providers share. Take notes if necessary, and don't hesitate to ask for clarification if something is unclear. Understanding your treatment options and their implications is key to making informed decisions.

- **Expressing Your Preferences:** Be assertive about your treatment preferences. If you believe in the benefits of an alkaline diet or specific supplements, share this with your team. Acknowledge any skepticism, but provide evidence or studies that support your approach.

3. Advocating for Yourself

- **Know Your Rights:** Understand your rights as a patient. You have the right to ask questions, seek second opinions, and refuse treatments that don't align with your values. Empower yourself by being informed about your treatment options and the potential outcomes.

- **Enlisting Support:** Bring a trusted friend or family member to appointments. They can help you remember details and provide emotional support. Having an advocate by your side can also reinforce your preferences to your healthcare team.

- **Documenting Your Journey:** Keep a detailed journal of your symptoms, treatment responses, and dietary changes. This record can be invaluable in discussions with your healthcare team, providing concrete evidence of how your approach is affecting your health.

4. Integrating Conventional and Alternative Treatments

- **Collaborative Care Plans:** Work with your healthcare team to create a care plan that incorporates both conventional treatments and your alkaline diet. Discuss how to schedule treatments in a way that allows you to maintain your nutritional regimen.

- **Monitoring Interactions:** Be aware of potential interactions between supplements and conventional treatments. Discuss these with your healthcare provider to ensure that your approach is safe and effective.

- **Staying Flexible:** Be open to adjusting your plan based on your body's responses. Cancer treatment can be unpredictable, so maintaining flexibility can help you adapt and make the best choices for your health.

5. Accessing Resources

- **Support Groups and Networks:** Look for local or online support groups for cancer patients. These can provide emotional support, shared experiences, and practical advice on navigating the healthcare system.

- **Educational Materials:** Utilize resources such as books, articles, and reputable websites to educate yourself about your condition, treatment options, and the benefits of an alkaline diet. Knowledge is a powerful tool in your healing journey.

- **Financial and Legal Assistance:** Investigate resources that can help with the financial aspects of cancer treatment, including insurance coverage, assistance programs, and legal rights concerning employment and healthcare.

Navigating the healthcare system can be daunting, but with the right tools and strategies, you can advocate for your needs and integrate your alkaline diet into your cancer treatment plan. Remember, you are your best advocate, and by building a strong healthcare team and communicating effectively, you can create a supportive environment that empowers your healing journey. Embrace your role in this process, and know that you have the strength to make informed decisions that align with your vision for health and wellness.

27 The Journey of Continuous Learning

In your quest to fight cancer naturally with an alkaline diet, one of the most empowering aspects is the commitment to lifelong learning. This chapter explores the importance of staying informed about nutrition, health, and the latest research related to cancer and holistic approaches.

1. Understanding the Evolving Landscape of Cancer Research

- **Stay Updated:** Cancer research is a rapidly evolving field. New studies and findings are released frequently, providing insights into treatment options, dietary impacts, and holistic health practices. Subscribing to reputable medical journals, newsletters, or websites can help you stay informed.

- **Follow Experts:** Identify experts in the field of oncology and nutrition who align with your beliefs. Many researchers and practitioners share valuable insights through blogs, social media, and webinars. Following their work can provide you with updated knowledge and inspiration.

2. Expanding Your Knowledge of Nutrition

- **Deepen Your Understanding of Alkaline Foods:** Explore the nutritional benefits of foods included in an alkaline diet. Research the vitamins, minerals, and phytochemicals that contribute to your health and how they interact with cancer treatment.

- **Experiment with New Recipes:** Cooking is an art, and trying new alkaline recipes can enhance your culinary skills while diversifying your diet. Experiment with different ingredients, cooking methods, and flavor combinations to keep your meals exciting and nutritious.

3. Engaging in Community Learning

- **Join Workshops and Classes:** Participating in cooking classes, nutrition workshops, or health seminars can provide hands-on learning experiences. Look for local community centers, health organizations, or online platforms that offer relevant programs.

- **Participate in Support Groups:** Engaging with others on similar journeys can foster a sense of community. Support groups often share valuable resources, tips, and personal experiences that can enhance your understanding and approach.

4. Integrating Mindfulness into Learning

- **Mindful Reflection:** Take time to reflect on what you learn. Keeping a journal can help you process new information, track your thoughts, and recognize how your understanding evolves over time.

- **Meditation and Mindfulness Practices:**
  Incorporating mindfulness techniques can
  enhance your learning experience. These
  practices can help you absorb information more
  effectively and cultivate a deeper connection with
  your journey.

5. Evaluating Your Progress

- **Set Learning Goals:** Establish personal learning
  objectives related to nutrition, health, and cancer
  treatment. These could include reading a certain
  number of articles per month, trying new recipes,
  or attending educational events.

- **Assessing Your Approach:** Periodically
  evaluate your dietary choices and overall health.
  Reflect on what has worked well and what
  adjustments might be necessary. This process can
  help you refine your approach and stay
  committed to your healing journey.

6. Connecting with Research Communities

- **Engage in Research Studies:** Consider
  participating in research studies or clinical trials
  that align with your interests. This not only
  contributes to the body of knowledge about
  cancer treatment but can also provide access to
  cutting-edge therapies and insights.

- **Collaborate with Researchers:** If you have a
  particular interest in a topic related to cancer and

nutrition, consider reaching out to researchers or institutions. They may welcome your interest and provide opportunities for collaboration or involvement.

The journey of fighting cancer naturally is not just about making dietary changes; it's about embracing a lifestyle of continuous learning and growth. By staying informed, connecting with others, and reflecting on your experiences, you empower yourself to make the best choices for your health. Remember, knowledge is not only a tool for healing but also a source of hope and resilience. Embrace the journey of learning, and let it guide you toward a healthier, more vibrant life.

28 The Future of Cancer Prevention and Treatment

The evolving field of dietary science shows promise in enhancing cancer prevention and treatment strategies. This chapter explores the potential for integrating alkaline diets into mainstream cancer care.

Evolving Dietary Science

1. Research Developments

- **Emerging Studies:** Ongoing research continues to investigate the links between diet, particularly alkaline diets, and cancer prevention. Studies indicate that diets rich in fruits and vegetables can play a role in reducing cancer risk.

2. Integrating Alkaline Diets into Mainstream Care

- **Clinical Trials:** Encouraging clinical trials are evaluating the effectiveness of dietary interventions, including alkaline diets, in cancer treatment protocols.

- **Educational Programs:** Healthcare systems are beginning to include dietary education in cancer treatment plans, emphasizing holistic approaches that incorporate nutrition.

3. Patient-Centric Care

- **Personalized Nutrition:** The future of cancer care may focus on personalized nutrition plans, allowing patients to choose dietary strategies that align with their health goals and preferences.

29 Embracing a Healthy Lifestyle Beyond Cancer

The Importance of Lifestyle Changes

After navigating through a cancer diagnosis and treatment, adopting a healthy lifestyle becomes crucial for long-term well-being and cancer prevention. While the focus during treatment may have been on immediate dietary and lifestyle adjustments, this chapter emphasizes the importance of maintaining those changes as part of a holistic approach to health.

Components of a Healthy Lifestyle

1. **Nutrition**: Continuing with an alkaline diet can help maintain optimal health. Focus on:

    o **Whole Foods**: Emphasize fresh fruits, vegetables, nuts, seeds, and whole grains.

    o **Limit Processed Foods**: Reduce consumption of processed and sugary foods to lower inflammation and promote overall health.

    o **Balanced Meals**: Create meals that include a variety of colors and nutrients to ensure a wide range of vitamins and minerals.

2. **Regular Exercise**: Physical activity is essential not just for physical health, but also for mental well-being.

   - **Types of Exercise**: Incorporate a mix of cardiovascular, strength, flexibility, and balance exercises. Activities like walking, swimming, yoga, and strength training can be beneficial.

   - **Set Realistic Goals**: Start with small, achievable goals to build confidence and consistency. Gradually increase the intensity and duration of your workouts.

3. **Hydration**: Staying well-hydrated is vital for overall health.

   - **Water Intake**: Aim for at least eight glasses of water a day. Alkaline water can be a beneficial addition, supporting hydration and balance.

   - **Limit Sugary Drinks**: Reduce or eliminate sodas and high-sugar beverages, opting instead for herbal teas or infused water for flavor.

4. **Mental and Emotional Health**: Prioritizing mental well-being is as crucial as physical health.

   - **Mindfulness Practices**: Incorporate mindfulness techniques such as meditation, deep breathing exercises, or journaling to reduce stress and promote emotional resilience.

- o **Therapy and Counseling**: Seeking professional help can provide support for emotional challenges and help process the experience of cancer.

5. **Sleep Hygiene**: Quality sleep is essential for healing and overall health.

- o **Establish a Routine**: Aim for 7-9 hours of sleep each night by establishing a consistent sleep schedule.

- o **Create a Sleep-Friendly Environment**: Keep your bedroom dark, quiet, and cool to promote restful sleep.

6. **Regular Check-ups**: After treatment, ongoing monitoring is vital.

- o **Follow-Up Appointments**: Schedule regular visits with your healthcare team to monitor your health and catch any potential issues early.

- o **Stay Informed**: Educate yourself about your health and remain proactive in discussing any changes or concerns with your medical team.

Building a Supportive Environment

1. **Engage Your Support Network**: Involve family and friends in your lifestyle changes. Cook healthy meals together, exercise as a group, or attend workshops on nutrition or wellness.

2. **Create a Positive Home Environment**: Fill your living space with healthy foods, motivational quotes, and reminders of your commitment to health.

3. **Stay Connected with Community Resources**: Join local health clubs, cooking classes, or wellness workshops to stay engaged and motivated.

Embracing a healthy lifestyle after cancer is not just about survival; it's about thriving. The choices you make today can significantly impact your long-term health and quality of life. By prioritizing nutrition, exercise, mental well-being, hydration, and regular check-ups, you are investing in your future and creating a foundation for lifelong health.

As you continue your journey, remember that every small step counts. Celebrate your progress, stay motivated, and keep learning about the ways to support your body and mind in achieving optimal health. Your experience has equipped you with the knowledge and resilience to live your healthiest life yet.

30 Building Your Support Network

Understanding the Importance of Support

Facing a cancer diagnosis can feel isolating, but having a strong support network can make a significant difference in your journey. Support systems provide emotional comfort, practical assistance, and resources for navigating both the medical landscape and the emotional challenges of cancer treatment.

Types of Support Networks

1. **Family and Friends**: Your immediate circle can be your greatest ally. They offer emotional support and can help with daily tasks like cooking, cleaning, or transportation to medical appointments. Open communication about your needs and feelings can strengthen these relationships.

2. **Cancer Support Groups**: Connecting with others who are going through similar experiences can be incredibly validating. Support groups provide a safe space to share fears, challenges, and triumphs. Many hospitals and community organizations offer these groups, both in-person and online.

3. **Healthcare Professionals**: Your medical team, including doctors, nurses, and nutritionists, plays a crucial role in your treatment. Don't hesitate to lean on them for advice, resources, and emotional

support. They can also help you find additional services, such as counseling or nutrition guidance.

4. **Online Communities**: The internet offers a wealth of resources and virtual support. Websites, forums, and social media groups dedicated to cancer support can provide information and connect you with others who share your journey.

5. **Holistic Practitioners**: Integrating alternative therapies can enhance your overall well-being. Practitioners of acupuncture, massage therapy, or yoga can provide additional support to manage stress and promote relaxation.

How to Build Your Support Network

1. **Identify Your Needs**: Consider what types of support would be most beneficial for you. Is it emotional support, practical help, or educational resources? Identifying your needs will help you reach out to the right people.

2. **Reach Out**: Don't be afraid to ask for help. Many people want to support you but may not know how. Share your feelings and needs with family and friends, and invite them to join you on this journey.

3. **Engage in Support Groups**: Look for local or online support groups focused on cancer. Many

groups are tailored to specific types of cancer or demographics, providing a community of shared experiences.

4. **Communicate Openly**: Keep your support network informed about your progress and challenges. Sharing your journey fosters deeper connections and encourages those around you to provide the support you need.

5. **Attend Workshops and Events**: Many organizations host workshops, seminars, and social events for cancer patients. These gatherings can provide valuable information and opportunities to meet others.

The Impact of a Strong Support Network

Having a robust support network can improve your emotional resilience, increase your motivation, and enhance your overall quality of life during treatment. Studies have shown that patients with strong support systems often experience better health outcomes and improved mental well-being.

As you navigate your cancer journey, remember that you are not alone. Building a support network takes time and effort, but the benefits are profound. Surround yourself with individuals who uplift and empower you, creating a community of strength and hope.

31 A Future of Hope and Healing

Reflecting on the Journey

As we arrive at the final chapter of this book, it's essential to reflect on the transformative journey we've embarked upon together. Fighting cancer, whether through conventional methods, an alkaline diet, or holistic approaches, requires not only courage and determination but also a strong foundation of knowledge and support. This chapter aims to encapsulate the key lessons learned and offer a vision of hope for the future.

The Power of Knowledge and Empowerment

1. **Understanding Cancer**: Knowledge about cancer, its mechanisms, and treatment options empowers you to make informed decisions about your health. By learning about the biology of cancer and the impact of lifestyle choices, you can take an active role in your healing journey.

2. **Adopting an Alkaline Diet**: The principles of an alkaline diet are not merely a fad; they represent a proactive approach to health. Embracing nutrient-rich foods can help create an environment in your body that is less hospitable to cancer cells. By prioritizing whole, unprocessed foods, you are choosing nourishment that supports your immune system and overall health.

3. **Holistic Practices**: Integrating mental, emotional, and physical health practices into your routine enriches your healing journey. Techniques such as mindfulness, yoga, and regular physical activity not only improve well-being but also foster resilience during difficult times.

Community and Support

1. **Building Your Support Network**: Surrounding yourself with a community of like-minded individuals can be a source of strength. Whether it's friends, family, support groups, or online communities, sharing experiences and resources can lighten the burden and foster connection.

2. **Advocacy and Awareness**: Becoming an advocate for cancer awareness and holistic health can provide purpose. Sharing your story, participating in fundraising events, or volunteering can help raise awareness and support for others facing similar challenges.

3. **Continual Learning**: The field of cancer research and holistic health is ever-evolving. Stay informed about new studies, treatments, and strategies for maintaining health. Engage with reliable resources, attend workshops, and connect with healthcare professionals who prioritize a comprehensive approach to cancer care.

A Vision for the Future

As you move forward, envision a life that is vibrant and fulfilling. The lessons learned through this journey can inform not only how you manage your health but also how you approach life itself. Consider these key takeaways:

1. **Embrace Change**: Change is a constant in life, and adapting to new circumstances is vital. Embrace the changes that come with a healthier lifestyle and remain open to exploring new avenues for growth.

2. **Cultivate Gratitude**: In the face of adversity, practicing gratitude can shift your perspective. Celebrate small victories and appreciate the support and love from those around you.

3. **Focus on Resilience**: Life may present challenges, but your ability to bounce back and learn from these experiences is what defines your strength. Cultivate resilience by nurturing a positive mindset and a strong support system.

Your Journey Continues

The journey of healing is ongoing, and while the road may have its ups and downs, the tools you've gained throughout this book are designed to support you every step of the way. Remember that you are not alone; your story can inspire and empower others. As you continue to fight for your health and well-being, may you carry with you the hope, strength, and knowledge to create a brighter future.

As you close this book, may it serve as a reminder of your incredible journey, the lessons learned, and the promise of a healthy, fulfilling life ahead. Together, we can advocate for a world where holistic health is embraced, and where individuals are empowered to fight cancer naturally and thrive.

EPILOGUE: Embracing the Journey Ahead

As we conclude this exploration of fighting cancer naturally with an alkaline diet, it's important to take a moment to reflect on the path you've traveled—both in reading this book and in your personal journey. The battle against cancer is not just a medical journey; it's a deeply personal and transformative experience that touches every aspect of life.

My ten-year journey of not knowing my cancer stage was incredibly stressful, but I'm grateful for the person who introduced me to alkaline water, leading to my research on alkaline diets. This approach worked for me and may help others with slow-growing or early-stage cancers. I recommend this lifestyle to everyone, as it promotes prevention and boosts energy.

The American Institute for Cancer Research estimates that diet and lifestyle changes could prevent a third of U.S. cancer cases, about 340,000 each year. Cancer remains the second leading cause of death in the U.S., following heart disease.

Though I've met college pre-med requirements and studied various health fields extensively, I am not a physician. Always consult a nutritionist, holistic doctor, or Doctor of Osteopathic Medicine (D.O.) before implementing any advice. Traditional doctors may focus on prescribing medication, but a more progressive practitioner might better align with these recommendations.

A Personal Commitment

You are equipped with knowledge, practical tools, and strategies that can empower you to take charge of your health. Adopting an alkaline diet is not just about dietary choices; it symbolizes a commitment to a lifestyle of wellness, resilience, and hope. This commitment extends beyond just nutrition; it encompasses a holistic approach to well-being—mind, body, and spirit.

The Power of Community

Remember that you are not alone in this fight. Building connections with others who share similar experiences can provide invaluable support. Whether it's through local support groups, online forums, or community organizations, these networks can foster a sense of belonging and understanding that can uplift your spirits during challenging times.

The Ongoing Journey

Healing is not a destination; it's an ongoing journey. As you integrate the principles of an alkaline diet and holistic health practices into your life, be open to learning and evolving. Every day presents new opportunities for growth, resilience, and healing. Celebrate your victories, no matter how small, and practice self-compassion during setbacks.

A Vision for the Future

As you move forward, envision a future filled with vitality, purpose, and joy. Armed with the insights from this book, you can make empowered choices that honor your body and support your overall health.

Embrace the power of knowledge and continue seeking information that resonates with you, whether it's new recipes, wellness practices, or scientific research.

I want to extend my heartfelt gratitude for allowing me to share this journey with you. Your willingness to explore natural methods of healing speaks to your strength and determination. Keep pushing forward, keep advocating for your health, and remember that hope is a powerful ally in this journey.

Together, let us foster a world where holistic health is recognized and celebrated, where individuals are empowered to take control of their well-being, and where every journey—yours included—leads to a brighter future

Thank you for reading my book and for being a part of this journey. May you find peace, healing, and joy in every step you take.

If you'd like a personalized meal plan or have questions, feel free to reach out at **fighting.cancer.naturally@gmail.com**.

Wishing you peace and health.

INTERESTING FACTS TO KNOW

Psychotropics and Nutrition

I believe many people prescribed psychotropics may not truly need them. America is a pill-pushing nation, evident in the substantial earnings of pharmaceutical sales representatives, who can make hundreds of thousands annually. This perspective is often unwelcome, as it challenges the interests of pharmaceutical companies and food producers like Nabisco.

I used to love Pepperidge Farm Milano cookies until I developed a gluten allergy, and I've noticed significant improvements in my health since cutting out processed and sugary foods. I've gotten sick less frequently, even while battling cancer.

Consider this: could some individuals diagnosed with depression or other mental illnesses simply have nutritional imbalances? Addressing these imbalances might reduce the need for psychotropics. For instance, people with autoimmune disorders related to iodine deficiency can experience mental health issues, which often improve when iodine levels are restored.

America's obesity epidemic correlates with rising mental illness rates. Obese individuals often face nutritional deficiencies, leading to unclear thinking. Exercise can improve mood and health, which is why it's prescribed for many health issues, including mental illness.

If we improved our diet, weight, and activity levels, could we reduce mental health issues and increase our lifespan? It's concerning that America ranks low in life expectancy, and our current habits contribute to this problem. Many companies benefit from this cycle, which complicates efforts to promote healthier living.

While synthetic medications serve important roles—like addressing shortages, providing controlled dosages, and offering quick relief—should we rely on them when natural solutions might suffice? Overuse of antibiotics and traces of psychotropic drugs in our water supply illustrate the urgency for regulation.

If we recognize cancer as a symptom of nutritional imbalance, why not consider mental illness similarly? A balanced diet could be a key to supporting our mental health. Just my two cents.

Aging and My Cancer Diet

At 43, many people mistakenly think I'm in my late 20s or early 30s, and I attribute this to my cancer diet. Following a quasi-vegan diet has transformed my skin and complexion, and I've noticed that my hair grows faster as well.

I feel more energetic now than I did as a teenager, even before my accident. Although I'm currently working through physical therapy to regain my flexibility, I'm optimistic about returning to my former self.

Americans Celebrate & Promote What Kills Them the Fastest

- Cigarette Smoke
- Marijuana Smoke
- Obesity and a Sedentary Lifestyle
- Fast Food
- Pork and Processed Meat
- Coke, Soda, and Carbonated Water
- Canned Food
- Sleeping Less than 6 Hours Nightly
- Alcohol
- Mind-Altering Street Drugs
- Misappropriated Pharmaceutical Drugs
- Potato Chips/French Fries
- Meat
- Refined Sugar and Candy

It's striking how we celebrate and promote habits that shorten our lifespans. Many seem to prefer the thrill of harmful choices over the commitment to living healthily. Ironically, most of these individuals would oppose assisted suicide laws, even while they engage in daily practices that lead them down a path of self-destruction.

While this book focuses on cancer, lupus has impacted many lives, and I've received questions about whether an alkaline diet can help those with lupus. I'm not a doctor, but I'll share what I've learned.

Lupus, or Systemic Lupus Erythematosus (SLE), along with Sjögren's syndrome and rheumatoid arthritis (RA), are autoimmune disorders typically treated with Plaquenil. Affecting around 5 million people worldwide, lupus can impact various systems, including the Central Nervous System, blood, joints, skin, and internal organs.

Inflammation and swelling are common issues associated with these disorders. An alkaline diet that eliminates refined sugars, alcohol, smoking, fried foods, unhealthy fats, sodium, red meat, gluten, and processed foods, combined with regular exercise, may help reduce inflammation and alleviate symptoms like fatigue, swelling, and joint pain.

People with lupus should avoid "nightshades"—such as eggplant, tomatoes, potatoes, and peppers—since these can worsen their condition. Nightshades belong to the Solanaceae family, which also includes tobacco. The glycoalkaloid solanine in potatoes and eggplants is known to increase inflammation and can aggravate conditions like Irritable Bowel Syndrome, Ulcerative Colitis, and Crohn's disease. Studies suggest that up to 70% of individuals with arthritis reported relief after eliminating nightshades from their diets.

Even though many nightshades are recognized for their cancer-fighting properties, they can provoke inflammation and should be avoided in a lupus-fighting diet.

Stay hydrated with plenty of water and consider drinking alkaline water with a pH of 9 or higher. If plain water is unappealing, enhance it with slices of lemon, lime, cucumber, or basil to improve flavor and raise pH levels. Always consult with your doctor or nutritionist before making significant dietary changes.

In general, avoid meat and focus on whole foods, such as fresh fruits, vegetables, nuts, and legumes that fall within the non-acidic range. It's also beneficial to find a natural sun protectant and ensure regular immunizations. For those with Sjögren's, incorporating flaxseed oil, glycerin tablets, and Vitamin E may promote moisture in the body. Additionally, stem cell transplants and treatments like rituximab could improve immune system functionality for patients who don't respond well to immunosuppressants.

Having lived with rheumatoid arthritis since I was eight, I also avoid nightshades. You may find value in exploring the effects of lectins, which are known to increase inflammation. Regular exercise is essential for managing both rheumatoid arthritis and lupus.

Here's to combating autoimmune disorders and cancer together! As always, consult a holistic doctor or nutritionist before making any major dietary changes.

Earlier, I mentioned my allergies to wheat, soy, quinoa, and nuts. These foods share a common factor: lectins.

Lectins are carbohydrate-binding proteins found in most plants, particularly in seeds and tubers like cereals, potatoes, and beans. Until recently, their main applications were in histology and blood transfusions. However, in the past two decades, we've come to recognize that many lectins can be toxic, inflammatory, or both. They are resistant to cooking and digestive enzymes, making them a potential source of "food poisoning."

Common Lectins:

Alkaline Lectins (generally less harmful):

- Cucumbers, Spinach
- Turnips
- Carrots, Avocados
- Sesame, Sunflower Seeds
- Purple & Sweet Potatoes
- Peas, Okra
- Asparagus, Pumpkins
- Lemons, Limes, Grapefruit

- Pomegranates

- Cherries, Tomatoes

- Bell Peppers

- Beets, Radish, Rhubarb

- Red Onions, Garlic

- Zucchini, Eggplant

- White Navy Beans, Lentils, Butter Beans, White Haricot Beans

- Quinoa, Buckwheat

- Soy Sprouts, Soybeans, Tofu

- Coconut

- Almonds, Almond Milk

Acidic Lectins (more problematic):

- Black Beans, Chickpeas

- Watermelon, Raspberries

- Blackberries, Blueberries

- Pineapples, Strawberries

- Oats, Wild Rice

- Cranberries, Cherries

- Bananas, Papaya, Grapes

- Oranges, Apples, Mango

- Wheat, Millet, Barley

- Walnuts, Hazelnuts

- Alcohol, Peanuts

- Cocoa, Coffee, Black Tea

- Soy Sauce, White Rice

- Mushrooms, Corn

- Bread, Yeast

- Eggs, Shellfish, Salmon

- Dairy, Cheese, Butter

Lectins can be particularly problematic for individuals with autoimmune disorders like rheumatoid arthritis, lupus, and Sjögren's syndrome, as they are inflammatory. Those with Irritable Bowel Syndrome (IBS) and heart disease may also be affected since lectins can bind to red blood cells, adhere to the intestinal lining or arteries, and potentially lead to conditions such as "leaky gut" or arterial blockages.

The intestinal lining is only one cell thick, so when lectins bind to it, they can cause damage, leading to "leaky gut syndrome." This is especially concerning if lectin-rich beans aren't cooked thoroughly, as cooking can deactivate lectins.

Lectins found in dairy, rice, bread, potatoes, and certain legumes, like cashews, almonds, pumpkin seeds, and soybeans, can trigger insatiable hunger pangs. This is relevant for those trying to lose weight, as they are often advised to avoid these foods.

The relationship between soybeans and thyroid function is controversial. Some, like Dr. Gundry, suggest that soy may disrupt thyroid function and promote overeating because it can prevent the brain from receiving hunger signals. However, according to the NIH, while soy foods may increase the thyroid hormone dosage needed by hypothyroid patients, they generally do not adversely affect thyroid function in healthy individuals.

As always, consult with a healthcare professional or nutritionist before making any significant dietary changes, especially if you have underlying health conditions.

Medical & Biological Terms

Alkaline:
Having properties of an alkali or containing alkali; specifically, a substance with a pH level greater than 7, which is considered basic or alkaline. Alkaline environments can neutralize acids and are found in various bodily fluids and substances.

Cachexia Cycle:
Cachexia, or wasting syndrome, involves significant weight loss, muscle atrophy, fatigue, weakness, and loss of appetite in individuals who are not actively trying to lose weight. It often occurs in people with chronic illnesses such as cancer, heart failure, or severe infections.

Cortisol:
A steroid hormone produced by the adrenal glands. It plays a critical role in regulating metabolism, immune responses, and the body's stress response by controlling blood sugar levels and reducing inflammation.

Epigenome:
A set of chemical modifications to the DNA and histone proteins in cells that regulate gene activity without altering the DNA sequence. These modifications can be influenced by environmental factors, diet, and stress, and they play a significant role in health, disease, and inheritance.

Immunotherapy:
A type of treatment that boosts or manipulates the immune system to help the body fight diseases, particularly cancer. It uses substances such as antibodies, cytokines, or vaccines to stimulate the body's natural defenses against disease.

IgE (Immunoglobulin E):
A type of antibody produced by the immune system in response to allergens. When IgE binds to allergens, it triggers the release of histamines and other chemicals, leading to allergic reactions such as inflammation, sneezing, or itching.

Krebs Cycle (Citric Acid Cycle):
A key metabolic pathway that occurs in the mitochondria of cells. It involves a series of chemical reactions that produce energy in the form of ATP by oxidizing acetyl-CoA derived from carbohydrates, fats, and proteins.

Macrophage:
A type of white blood cell that engulfs and digests cellular debris, foreign substances, and pathogens. Macrophages play a critical role in the immune response by helping to eliminate infection and stimulate other immune cells.

Melatonin:
A hormone produced by the pineal gland in the brain. It regulates sleep-wake cycles and circadian rhythms. Melatonin production is typically triggered by darkness,

and supplements are sometimes used to help with sleep
disorders.

Mesothelioma:
A type of cancer that affects the mesothelium, a
protective lining of the lungs, abdomen, heart, and other
organs. Mesothelioma is most commonly associated with
asbestos exposure.

Metastatic (Metastasis):
Refers to cancer that has spread from the primary site
where it originated to other parts of the body. Metastatic
cancer cells can invade nearby tissues and form new
tumors in distant organs.

Natural Killer (NK) Cells:
A type of lymphocyte (a subtype of white blood cells)
that plays a crucial role in the body's defense against
tumors and virally infected cells. NK cells recognize and
destroy compromised cells without the need for prior
exposure to the pathogen.

Nagalase:
A protein produced by cancer cells and certain viruses,
including HIV and hepatitis. Nagalase inhibits the
immune system by disrupting the production of GcMAF,
a protein that activates macrophages to destroy cancer
cells.

Pulmonary:
Related to or affecting the lungs and respiratory system.
Pulmonary diseases include conditions like asthma,

bronchitis, pneumonia, and chronic obstructive
pulmonary disease (COPD).

Pharmacological & Chemical Terms

Chelation:
A medical procedure that involves the use of chelating agents, which bind to heavy metals like lead, mercury, and arsenic, to remove them from the body. Chelation therapy is often used in cases of heavy metal poisoning.

EDTA (Ethylenediamine tetra-acetic acid):
A chemical compound used in chelation therapy to bind and remove heavy metals from the bloodstream. It is also used in various industrial and scientific applications to prevent metal ion contamination.

Psychotropic:
A term referring to substances that affect the mind, emotions, or behavior. Psychotropic drugs are commonly used to treat mental health conditions, such as depression, anxiety, and schizophrenia, by altering brain chemistry.

THC (Tetrahydrocannabinol):
The principal psychoactive compound in cannabis, responsible for the euphoric "high" associated with marijuana use. THC interacts with the brain's endocannabinoid system, influencing mood, appetite, and memory.

Environmental & Industrial Terms

Asbestos:
A naturally occurring fibrous silicate mineral that is resistant to heat, fire, and chemicals. Historically used in

construction and manufacturing, asbestos exposure is now known to cause serious health risks, including lung cancer and mesothelioma.

Therapeutic & Health-Related Terms

Cannabis:

A plant used both for its fiber (hemp) and its psychoactive properties (marijuana). Cannabis contains compounds like THC and CBD, which are used recreationally and medicinally to treat pain, anxiety, and certain neurological conditions.

Six Sigma Lean Standard:

A data-driven approach to process improvement, Six Sigma aims to reduce defects and improve efficiency in any organizational process. Lean principles focus on eliminating waste and optimizing workflows to achieve high-quality results with minimal resources.

Miscellaneous Terms

Serotonin:

A neurotransmitter that plays a key role in regulating mood, emotions, and sleep. Low levels of serotonin are associated with depression, while high levels contribute to feelings of well-being and happiness.

Bibliography

American Cancer Society. (2016). *Microwaves, Radiowaves, and Other Types of Radiofrequency Radiation.* Retrieved from https://www.cancer.org/cancer/cancer-causes/radiation-exposure/radiofrequency-radiation.html

American Cancer Society. (2014). *Anti-Perspirants and Breast Cancer Risk.* Retrieved from https://www.cancer.org/cancer/cancer-causes/antiperspirants-and-breast-cancer-risk.html

American Cancer Society. (2015). *Asbestos and Cancer Risk.* Retrieved from https://www.cancer.org/cancer/cancer-causes/asbestos.html

American Lung Association. (2015). *Marijuana and Lung Health.* Retrieved from http://www.lung.org/stop-smoking/smoking-facts/marijuana-and-lung-health.html

Batts, V. (2016). *Colgate Toothpaste Found to Contain Cancer-Causing Chemical.* World Health. Retrieved from https://www.worldhealth.net/forum/topic/3665/

Be Well Coaching Weblog. (2013). *Can Eating Healthfully Hurt? Oxalate Consumption and Pain.* Retrieved from https://bewellcoaching.wordpress.com/2013/05/28/can-eating-healthfully-hurt-oxalate-consumption-and-pain/

British Journal of Cancer. (2012). *Asbestos and Shift Work Boost Work-Related Cancer Deaths to Over 8,000 a Year.* Cancer Research UK. Retrieved from https://www.cancerresearchuk.org/about-us/cancer-news/press-release/2012-06-20-asbestos-and-shift-work-boost-work-related-cancer-deaths-to-over-8000-a-year

Cancer Council NSW. (2012). *Microwave Ovens Do Not Cause Cancer.* Retrieved from https://www.cancercouncil.com.au/86089/cancer-information/general-information-cancer-information/cancer-questions-myths/environmental-and-occupational-carcinogens/microwave-ovens-do-not-cause-cancer/

Cancer Journal. (2015). *Mindfulness-Based Cancer Recovery and Supportive Expressive Therapy Maintain Telomere Length Relative to Controls in Distressed Breast Cancer Survivors.* Retrieved from http://onlinelibrary.wiley.com/doi/10.1002/cncr.29063/full

Cancer Prevention Research and Men's Health. (2011). *Do Eggs Cause Prostate Cancer?* Retrieved from https://www.menshealth.com/health/do-eggs-cause-prostate-cancer

Centers for Disease Control and Prevention (CDC). (2017). *Short Sleep Duration Among US Adults.* Retrieved from https://www.cdc.gov/sleep/data_statistics.html

Davis, N. (2016). *Toxic Chemicals in Household Dust Linked to Cancer and Infertility.* The Guardian. Retrieved from https://www.theguardian.com/science/2016/sep/14/toxic-chemicals-household-dust-health-cancer-infertility

Garcia, C. (2012). *Cancer is a Symptom: The Real Cause Revealed.* Utopia Wellness. Retrieved from https://utopiawellness.com/cancer-is-a-symptom/

Great Life Global. *All About Nightshades.* Retrieved from http://www.greatlifeglobal.com/services/health-a-wellness-consultations/29.html

FAU.edu. (2013). *How Society's Light Pollution Affects Human Breast Cancer.* Retrieved from http://cescos.fau.edu/observatory/lightpol-BrCa.html

Hamaguchi R, Isowa M, Narui R, Morikawa H, Wada H. Clinical review of alkalization therapy in cancer treatment. Front Oncol. 2022 Sep 14;12:1003588. doi: 10.3389/fonc.2022.1003588. PMID: 36185175; PMCID: PMC9516301 Retrieved from: Clinical review of alkalization therapy in cancer treatment - PMC (nih.gov)

Helio. (2018). *High Costs Drive Underuse of Brachytherapy for Cervical Cancer.* Journals Plus. Retrieved from https://www.healio.com/hematology-oncology/gynecologic-cancer/news/in-the-journals/%7Bcd77b6a5-49c0-405f-ac69-0b3fc896f39f%7D/high-costs-drive-underuse-of-brachytherapy-for-cervical-cancer

International Journal of Epidemiology. (2009). *Risk of Cancer Among Hairdressers and Related Workers: A Meta-Analysis.* Retrieved from https://academic.oup.com/ije/article/38/6/1512/672312

Kentish, B. (2017). *Additive Found in Toothpaste and Food Products Could Cause Cancer, Say Scientists.* The Independent. Retrieved from https://www.independent.co.uk/news/science/toothpaste-additive-e171-titanium-dioxide-food-products-cancer-cause-scientists-a7541956.html

Kozlowska, R., et al. (2016). *Association Between Cancer and Allergies.* Journal of Epidemiology. Retrieved from https://www.ncbi.nlm.nih.gov/pmc/articles/PMC4982132/

Libereros, S., et al. (2015). *Allergen-Induced Pulmonary Inflammation Enhances Mammary Tumor Growth and Metastasis: Role of CHI3LI.* Journal of Leukocyte Biology. Retrieved from https://citeseerx.ist.psu.edu/viewdoc/download?doi=10.1.1.884.173&rep=rep1&type=pdf

Maidhof, W. (2012). *Lupus: An Overview of the Disease and Management Options.* NIH. Retrieved from https://www.ncbi.nlm.nih.gov/pmc/articles/PMC3351863/

Martin, R. K. (2014). *Mast Cell Histamine Promotes the Immunoregulatory Activity of Myeloid-Derived*

Suppressor Cells. Journal of Leukocyte Biology. Retrieved from https://www.ncbi.nlm.nih.gov/pmc/articles/PMC4056279/

Martínez-Piñeiro JA, Jiménez León J, Martínez-Piñeiro L Jr, Fiter L, Mosteiro JA, Navarro J, García Matres MJ, Cárcamo P. Bacillus Calmette-Guerin versus doxorubicin versus thiotepa: a randomized prospective study in 202 patients with superficial bladder cancer. J Urol. 1990 Mar;143(3):502-6. doi: 10.1016/s0022-5347(17)40002-4. PMID: 2106041. Retrieved from: Bacillus Calmette-Guerin versus doxorubicin versus thiotepa: a randomized prospective study in 202 patients with superficial bladder cancer - PubMed (nih.gov)

Mayo Clinic. (2016). *Iron Deficiency Anemia.* Retrieved from https://www.mayoclinic.org/diseases-conditions/iron-deficiency-anemia/symptoms-causes/syc-20355034

Mercola.com. (2013). *The Benefits of Ketogenic Diet and Its Role in Cancer Treatments.* Retrieved from https://articles.mercola.com/sites/articles/archive/2013/06/16/ketogenic-diet-benefits.aspx

Mittelman SD. The Role of Diet in Cancer Prevention and Chemotherapy Efficacy. Annu Rev Nutr. 2020 Sep 23;40:273-297. doi: 10.1146/annurev-nutr-013120-041149. Epub 2020 Jun 16. PMID: 32543948; PMCID: PMC8546934. Retrieved from: The Role of Diet in

Cancer Prevention and Chemotherapy Efficacy - PMC (nih.gov)

National Cancer Institute. *Psychological Stress and Cancer.* Retrieved from https://www.cancer.gov/about-cancer/coping/feelings/stress-fact-sheet

New York Times. (2017). *A Host of Ills When Iron's Out of Balance.* Retrieved from https://well.blogs.nytimes.com/2012/08/13/a-host-of-ills-when-irons-out-of-balance/

New York Times. (2017). *The Chemicals in Your Mac and Cheese.* Retrieved from https://www.nytimes.com/2017/07/12/well/eat/the-chemicals-in-your-mac-and-cheese.html

New York State Department of Health. (2016). *Exposure to Smoke from Fires.* Retrieved from https://www.health.ny.gov/environmental/outdoors/air/smoke_from_fire.htm

O'Connor, A. (2013). *Really? The Claim: Fresh Produce Has More Nutrients Than Canned.* The New York Times. Retrieved from https://well.blogs.nytimes.com/2013/05/27/really-the-claim-fresh-produce-has-more-nutrients-than-canned/

Pascale RM, Calvisi DF, Simile MM, Feo CF, Feo F. The Warburg Effect 97 Years after Its Discovery. Cancers (Basel). 2020 Sep 30;12(10):2819. doi: 10.3390/cancers12102819. PMID: 33008042; PMCID:

PMC7599761. Retrieved from: The Warburg Effect 97 Years after Its Discovery - PubMed (nih.gov)

PBS. (2017). *Common House Dust Could Contain Cancer-Causing Molecules.* Retrieved from https://www.pbs.org/wgbh/nova/next/body/dust-cancer/

Petre, A. (2016). *Lemon Juice: Acidic or Alkaline and Does It Matter?* Healthline. Retrieved from https://www.healthline.com/nutrition/lemon-juice-acidic-or-alkaline

PubMed. (2011). *Exercise Lowers Estrogen and Progesterone Levels in Perimenopausal Women at High Risk of Breast Cancer.* Retrieved from https://www.ncbi.nlm.nih.gov/m/pubmed/21903887/

Pyo, Y. H., et al. (2014). *Comparison of the Effects of Blending and Juicing of the Phytochemicals Contents and the Antioxidant Capacity of Typical Kernel Korean Fruit Juices.* NIH. Retrieved from https://www.ncbi.nlm.nih.gov/pmc/articles/PMC4103735/

Rondavelli, M., et al. (2013). *Update on the Role of Melatonin in the Prevention of Tumorigenesis and in the Management of Cancer Correlates, Such as Sleep-Wake and Mood Disturbances: Review and Remarks.* Retrieved from https://link.springer.com/content/pdf/10.1007/s40520-013-0118-6.pdf

Ruvulo-Wilkes, V. (2017). *Can Cancer Cause Iron Deficiency in the Blood?* LiveStrong. Retrieved from https://www.livestrong.com/article/411382-can-cancer-cause-an-iron-deficiency-in-blood/

Rybnikova, N. A., et al. (2016). *Does Artificial Light-at-Night Exposure Contribute to the Worldwide Obesity Pandemic?* International Journal of Obesity. Retrieved from
https://www.ncbi.nlm.nih.gov/m/pubmed/26795746/

RXAir. (2015). *Protect Cancer Patients with UV Light Air Purifiers.* Retrieved from https://www.rxair.com/protect-cancer-patients-with-uv-light-air-purifiers/

Safer Chemicals.org. (2016). *New Report Shows Big Retailers Cracking Down on Toxic Chemicals in Consumer Products But Others Remain Serious Laggards.* Retrieved from
https://saferchemicals.org/newsroom/new-report-shows-big-retail

Schwalfenberg GK. The alkaline diet: is there evidence that an alkaline pH diet benefits health? J Environ Public Health. 2012;2012:727630. doi: 10.1155/2012/727630. Epub 2011 Oct 12. PMID: 22013455; PMCID: PMC3195546. Retrieved from: The Alkaline Diet: Is There Evidence That an Alkaline pH Diet Benefits Health? - PMC (nih.gov)

Singh DN, Bohra JS, Dubey TP, Shivahre PR, Singh RK, Singh T, Jaiswal DK. Common foods for boosting human immunity: A review. Food Sci Nutr. 2023 Aug 18;11(11):6761-6774. doi: 10.1002/fsn3.3628. PMID: 37970422; PMCID: PMC10630845. Retrieved from: Common foods for boosting human immunity: A review - PMC (nih.gov)

Stromsnes K, Correas AG, Lehmann J, Gambini J, Olaso-Gonzalez G. Anti-Inflammatory Properties of Diet: Role in Healthy Aging. Biomedicines. 2021 Jul 30;9(8):922. doi: 10.3390/biomedicines9080922. PMID: 34440125; PMCID: PMC8389628. Retrieved from: Anti-Inflammatory Properties of Diet: Role in Healthy Aging - PMC (nih.gov)

Wada, H., Morikawa, H., Hamaguchi, R. Narui, R. Can Alkaline Diet Improve Cancer Outcomes? 2020 March 4. doi: 10.33548/SCIENTIA483 Retrieved from: Dr Hiromi Wada - Can an Alkaline Diet Improve Cancer Outcomes? • scientia.global

NOTES

1. Cancer and Heart Disease Statistics:

- CDC Compendium

- CDC Fast Stats

2. Sleep Studies:

- **European Heart Journal Excerpt**: "Consistently sleeping less than six hours a night nearly doubles your risk of heart attack and stroke, according to a review of 15 studies published in the European Heart Journal. Another study found that consistently sleep-deprived people were 12 percent more likely to die over the 25-year study period than those who got six to eight hours of sleep a night."

  - Tips from the National Sleep Foundation:

    1. Make the room pitch-black dark, and set the thermostat between 60 and 67 degrees.

    2. Exercise daily, but not close to bedtime.

    3. Stick to a regular sleep schedule.

    4. Shut down electronics an hour before bed.

5. Replace your mattress if it's over 10 years old.

Sleep Study References:

Watson NF, Badr MS, Belenky G, et al. Consensus statement on the recommended amount of sleep for a healthy adult. *Sleep* 2015;38:1161-1183.

Zhang X, Holt JB, Lu H, et al. Multilevel regression for small area estimation of chronic obstructive pulmonary disease prevalence using BRFSS. *Am J Epidemiol* 2014;179(8):1025-1033.

Paruthi S, Brooks LJ, D'Ambrosio C, et al. Recommended amount of sleep for pediatric populations: *J Clin Sleep Med* 2016;12(6):785–786.

Wheaton AG, Olsen EO, Miller GF, Croft JB. Sleep duration and injury-related risk behaviors among high school students — United States, 2007–2013. *MMWR Morb Mortal Wkly Rep* 2016;65:337–341.

3. Ways to Live Longer:

- AARP's 50 Ways to Live Longer

4. Body Iron and Cancer Risk:

- **Iron Storage**: Iron is stored, mostly in the liver, as ferritin or hemosiderin. Ferritin can hold about 4500 iron ions per molecule.

  - Iron Storage

- **Cancer Risk**:

    - Body Iron Stores and the Risk of Cancer

5. Antiperspirants and Cancer:

- Cancer.org on Antiperspirants and Breast Cancer Risk

6. Brachytherapy for Cervical Cancer:

- Underuse Due to High Costs

7. Allergy and Cancer References:

Mills PK, Beeson WL, Fraser GE, Phillips RL. *Allergy and Cancer: Organ Site-Specific Results from the Adventist Health Study. American Journal of Epidemiology*, Volume 136, Issue 3, August 1992, Pages 287–295.
DOI link

8. Alkaline Diet References:

Schwalfenberg, G. *The Alkaline Diet: Is There Evidence That an Alkaline pH Diet Benefits Health? Journal of Environmental and Public Health*, 2011.
Article link

9. Oxalates References:

- NutritionFacts: Hazards of Oxalates

- Oxalates and Muscle Pain

10. Immunotherapy References:

Aldeghi R, Lissoni P, Barni S, et al. *Low-dose interleukin-2 subcutaneous immunotherapy in association with melatonin as first-line therapy for hepatocellular carcinoma. Eur J Cancer* 1994;30A:167-170. [PubMed link]

11. Rural Health Risks:

- CDC: Rural Death Risk

This structure organizes the topics clearly by subject and provides links and references where applicable.

4o

References About Marijuana and Health:

1. **American Lung Association**:

    o   "Marijuana and Lung Health"

    o   Marijuana and Lung Health

    o   (2015)

2. **National Institute on Drug Abuse**:

    o   DrugFacts: Marijuana

    o   Volkow ND, Baler RD, Compton WM, Weiss SRB.

    o   Adverse health effects of marijuana use.

    o   *N Engl J Med.* 2014;370(23):2219-27.

3. **Pediatric Marijuana Exposures**:

- o Wang GS, Roosevelt G, Heard K.

- o Pediatric marijuana exposures in a medical marijuana state.

- o *JAMA Pediatr.* 2013;167(7):630-3.

4. **Marijuana Smoking and Lung Health**:

- o Tashkin DP.

- o Effects of marijuana smoking on the lung.

- o *Ann Am Thorac Soc.* 2013;10(3):239-47.

5. **Comparing Marijuana and Tobacco Smoke**:

- o Moir D, Rickert WS, Levasseur G, et al.

- o A comparison of mainstream and sidestream marijuana and tobacco cigarette smoke produced under two machine smoking conditions.

- o *Chem Res Toxicol.* 2008;21(2):494-502. doi:10.1021/tx700275p.

6. **Neutral Components in Marijuana and Tobacco Smoke**:

- o Novotny M, Merli F, Wiesler D, Fencl M, Saeed T.

- o Fractionation and capillary gas chromatographic—mass spectrometric characterization of the neutral components in marijuana and tobacco smoke condensates.

- o *J Chromatogr A.* 1982;238:141-50. doi: 10.1016/S0021-9673(00)82720-X.

7. **Carcinogenicity of Marijuana Smoke**:

- o Hoffmann D, Brunnemann KD, Gori GB, Wynder EL.

- o On the Carcinogenicity of Marijuana Smoke.

- o In: Runeckles VC, ed.

- o *Recent Advances in Phytochemistry.* Springer US; 1975:63-81.

8. **Pulmonary Hazards of Smoking Marijuana Compared to Tobacco**:

- o Wu T-C, Tashkin DP, Djahed B, Rose JE.

- o Pulmonary hazards of smoking marijuana as compared with tobacco.

- o *N Engl J Med.* 1988;318(6):347-51.

9. **Pulmonary Effects of Marijuana Inhalation**:

- o Howden ML, Naughton MT.

- o Pulmonary effects of marijuana inhalation.

- *Expert Rev Respir Med.* 2011;5(1):87-92.

10. **Health Care Use by Frequent Marijuana Smokers**:

- Polen MR, Sidney S, Tekawa IS, Sadler M, Friedman GD.

- Health care use by frequent marijuana smokers who do not smoke tobacco.

- *West J Med.* 1993;158(6):596-601.

Excerpt About Phthalates in Kraft Macaroni and Cheese:

- **Author**: Roni Caryn Rabin

- **Date**: July 12, 2017

- **Summary**:

  - Phthalates, harmful chemicals linked to male hormone disruption, genital birth defects, and learning/behavioral problems in children, are still found in high concentrations in Kraft macaroni and cheese mixes made with powdered cheese.

  - These chemicals, banned from children's toys over a decade ago, are not banned in food, despite their migration from packaging and manufacturing equipment.

- o A study of 30 cheese products found phthalates in all but one sample, with the highest levels in processed cheese powder. Organic varieties were not exempt.

- o Advocacy groups such as the Environmental Health Strategy Center, Ecology Center, Healthy Babies Bright Futures, and Safer States funded the report.

- o The study has not yet been peer-reviewed.

Excerpt About Cervical Cancer Treatment from VeryWell.com

Source: VeryWell.com: Cervical Dysplasia

Overview

- **Connection between HPV and Cervical Dysplasia**: HPV (Human Papillomavirus), a virus transmitted through sexual contact, is strongly linked to cervical dysplasia. For most women, both HPV and cervical dysplasia resolve on their own without treatment. However, in some cases, untreated HPV can lead to severe cervical changes and eventually cervical cancer.

- **Risk Factors:**

- o Smoking accelerates the effects of HPV on the cervix, increasing the risk of developing cervical dysplasia and cervical cancer.

  - o Other risk factors include being HIV positive, having multiple sexual partners, and giving birth before age 20.

Diagnosis

- **Pap Test**: Cervical dysplasia is typically diagnosed via a Pap test, where cervical cells are collected for lab analysis. If abnormal cells are detected, an HPV test may be performed.

- **ASC-US (Atypical Squamous Cells of Uncertain Significance)**: If atypical cells are detected, a repeat test in 12 months is usually recommended. A biopsy may be required if HPV is present or if abnormal cells are found again.

  - o **Colposcopy**: During this procedure, a biopsy is performed to check for precancerous cells, known as cervical intraepithelial neoplasia (CIN). CIN is graded as follows:

    - CIN 1: Mild dysplasia

    - CIN 2: Moderate dysplasia

    - CIN 3: Severe dysplasia or carcinoma in situ (pre-cancerous)

Treatment

- **CIN 1**: This grade is usually monitored with regular Pap tests and HPV screenings, without immediate treatment.

- **CIN 2 & 3**: More severe dysplasia requires treatment to remove abnormal cells to prevent cancer. Treatment options include:

  - **Cryosurgery**: Freezing abnormal tissue using a frozen probe.

  - **LEEP (Loop Electrosurgical Excision Procedure)**: Uses an electrically charged wire to remove tissue.

  - **Laser Surgery**: Abnormal tissue is treated using a carbon dioxide laser.

  - **Cold Knife Cone Biopsy**: Uses a scalpel to surgically remove tissue.

  - Local anesthesia is commonly used during these procedures, which are usually performed as outpatient surgeries.

- **Post-Treatment Recurrence**: The recurrence rate of CIN is around 5.3% for women treated with cryosurgery or LEEP and 1.4% for those treated with cold knife conization, although cold knife procedures may have a slightly higher complication rate.

Follow-Up

- Regular monitoring is required following treatment. If abnormal cells return, additional treatment may be needed. Since HPV infections can persist, there is an ongoing risk of abnormal tissue developing later.

Coping

- Receiving a diagnosis of cervical dysplasia can be frightening, but following up with recommended treatments and monitoring reduces the likelihood of cancer progression.

Sources:

- Hoffman, S., Le, T., Lockhart, A., et al. "Patterns of Persistent HPV Infection After Treatment for Cervical Intraepithelial Neoplasia (CIN): A Systematic Review." *International Journal of Cancer*, 2017.

- Santesso, N., Mustafa, R., Wiercioch, W., et al. "Systematic Reviews and Meta-Analysis."

References About Juicing

- National Institutes of Health: Juicing

References About Psychotropics, Neurology, and Nutrition

1. EurekaAlert: Nutrition in Psychiatric Treatment

2. Psychiatry Advisor: Importance of Nutrition in Psychiatric Treatment

3. MD Edge: Vitamin Deficiencies and Mental Health

4. NCBI Books: Nutrition and Mental Health

References for CNS Lupus

- Lupus Rebel: What is Lupus?
    - Affects an estimated 5 million people worldwide.
    - SLE (Systemic Lupus Erythematosus) can involve the skin, joints, internal organs, and the nervous system.
- This Lupus Life: The Alkaline Diet for Autoimmunity
- Medscape: CNS Lupus Overview

CNS Lupus Overview

- **Author**: Tarakad S Ramachandran, MBBS, MBA, MPH, FAAN, FACP, FAHA, FRCP, FRCPC, FRS, LRCP, MRCP, MRCS

- **Chief Editor**: Niranjan N Singh, MBBS, MD, DM, FAHS, FAANEM

- **Updated**: August 22, 2017

Background

- Neurologic manifestations are a feature of SLE, a multisystem autoimmune connective tissue disorder with various clinical presentations. It can affect the central and peripheral nervous systems and muscles.

- CNS lupus is serious but potentially treatable. It presents significant diagnostic challenges and is often part of the differential diagnosis for many neurologic conditions. Patients with SLE may initially present with neurologic symptoms before being diagnosed.

Diagnostic Imaging

- An axial T2-weighted MRI shows ischemia in the right periventricular white matter of a 41-year-old woman with longstanding SLE. Symptoms included headache and subtle cognitive impairments, but no motor deficits were noted.

Pathophysiology

- The pathophysiology of SLE is not fully defined. Genetic factors, particularly human leukocyte antigens (HLA), may increase susceptibility, though environmental triggers are also likely involved.

- Certain medications can induce drug-induced lupus, which differs from classic SLE. The autoimmune reaction in SLE affects multiple sites through mechanisms like immune complex deposition and direct autoantibody attacks.

- Non-neurologic damage can occur in areas such as the kidneys, joints, pleura, pericardium, skin, cardiac and vascular endothelium, and mucosal tissues.

Etiology of Neurologic Manifestations in Systemic Lupus Erythematosus (SLE)

1. Organic Encephalopathies

- The most common neurologic manifestation of SLE is organic encephalopathy, a diffuse syndrome poorly correlated with the extent of vasculitis or thromboembolism.

- Functional imaging studies, such as PET, functional MRI, or SPECT, demonstrate patchy areas of dysfunction that are not visible on conventional MRI. This suggests a metabolic alteration independent of cerebral blood flow obstruction.

- The mechanism behind these metabolic alterations remains unknown.

2. Vasculitis and Vasculopathy

- Histological studies of apparent vasculitis show degenerative changes in small vessel walls with minimal or no inflammatory infiltrates.

- Chronic immune complex deposition and cytokine-mediated effects are potential mechanisms for SLE vasculopathy.

- Inflammatory and non-inflammatory SLE vasculopathies may be indistinguishable, and terms like "cerebritis" and "vasculitis" are commonly used, though evolving understanding may eventually refine these concepts.

3. Large- and Medium-Sized Vessel Involvement

- In addition to small vessel vasculopathy, inflammatory changes can occur in larger vessels, leading to classic vasculitis, which may result in clinical stroke syndromes due to local thrombosis or artery-to-artery emboli.

- Stroke etiologies in SLE may also include local thrombosis from antiphospholipid antibodies, affecting small and medium-sized arteries, veins, or venous sinuses.

4. Libman-Sacks Endocarditis (LSE)

- LSE is a sterile endocardial inflammation producing vegetations on the heart valves, more frequently seen in patients with antiphospholipid antibodies.

- LSE can cause diffuse microembolization, clinically similar to vasculitis or cerebritis, and in focal clinical syndromes, cardiac emboli are often more responsible than vasculitic or thrombotic processes.

5. Antiphospholipid Antibodies

- These antibodies are associated with several complications, including LSE, local arterial or venous thrombosis, hemorrhagic diathesis, myelopathy, and non-neurologic manifestations like spontaneous abortion.

- Dural sinus thrombosis, a rare complication of SLE-associated hypercoagulability, is often linked with antiphospholipid antibodies. This can be imaged through MRI, MR venous angiography, conventional angiography, or radionuclide brain scans.

Drug-Induced Myopathies in SLE

1. Steroid-Induced Myopathy

- Steroid-induced myopathy is the most common form, characterized by progressing painless muscle weakness, fatigue, and atrophy. This occurs due to glucocorticoid use, with fluorinated glucocorticoids having a higher risk.

- Muscle biopsy shows slight fiber size variation, type 2b fiber atrophy, minimal or no fiber necrosis, and no inflammatory cells. There may also be slight myofibrillar loss with glycogen and lipid accumulation.

---

2. Amphiphilic Drug Myopathies

- Drugs with hydrophobic and hydrophilic regions, like chloroquine and hydroxychloroquine, can cause multisystem disorders, including neuropathy, myopathy, and cardiomyopathy.

- Amphiphilic drugs can cause vacuolar myopathy, especially with a 500 mg daily dose of chloroquine for over a year.

- Muscle biopsy reveals vacuoles containing lipid and membranous material, with acid phosphatase staining in muscle fibers and normal PAS staining for glycogen.

Epidemiology of Neuropsychiatric Systemic Lupus Erythematosus (NPSLE)

1. Definition and Classification

- NPSLE syndromes are defined by the American College of Rheumatology (ACR) with 19 specific diagnostic criteria.

- Less than 40-50% of NPSLE events are attributed to underlying CNS lupus activity (primary NPSLE).

- The remaining events are indirectly associated with SLE, resulting from metabolic disturbances, infections, or drug effects (secondary NPSLE).

---

2. Prevalence

- Data from large cohorts indicate a prevalence rate of approximately 30–40% for NPSLE.

- NPSLE appears to be equally common in children and adults.

---

3. Clinical Findings

- A three-year prospective study involving 370 SLE patients with no prior CNS involvement found that clinically severe CNS involvement is rare, occurring at a rate of 7.8 per 100 person-years.

Prognosis of Neuropsychiatric Events in SLE

1. Outcomes

- CNS-specific statistics are limited; however, neuropsychiatric events due to SLE generally have a more favorable outcome compared to those secondary to non-SLE causes.

- SLE-related events typically occur early in the illness, impacting the patient's quality of life with varying severity and frequency.

2. Impact of Neurologic Complications

- Neurologic complications can worsen prognosis, particularly when associated with refractory seizures, encephalopathy, or paralysis due to stroke or myelopathy.

- Taddio et al. found that atypical manifestations of pediatric SLE at presentation and early kidney disease correlate with poorer outcomes.

Similarly, kidney and CNS diseases during follow-up were associated with worse prognoses.

References About Lectins

1. General Information

- Lectins are ubiquitous in nature and found in many foods.

- Certain foods, like beans and grains, need to be cooked or fermented to reduce lectin content, but those consumed in a balanced diet are generally not harmful.

- Some lectins, such as CLEC11A, promote bone growth, while others, like ricin, are potent toxins.

---

2. Mechanism of Action

- Lectins can be disabled by specific mono- and oligosaccharides that bind to them, preventing their attachment to cell membrane carbohydrates.

- Their selectivity makes them useful for blood type analysis and in genetically engineered crops for pest and herbicide resistance.

---

3. Food Sources of Lectins

- **Grains**: Wheat (including wheat germ), barley, corn, rice, oats, buckwheat, rye, millet.

- **Legumes**: Various types of beans and pulses.

- **Fruits and Vegetables**: Tomatoes, potatoes, sweet potatoes, zucchini, carrots, beets, mushrooms, asparagus, cucumbers, citrus fruits (oranges, lemons), berries (blackberries, strawberries), and other fruits (pomegranate, grapes, cherries, bananas, etc.).

- **Nuts and Seeds**: Walnuts, hazelnuts, peanuts, sunflower seeds, sesame seeds.

- **Other Foods**: Chocolate, coffee, and certain spices (caraway, nutmeg, peppermint, garlic).